HEMODYNAMICS.

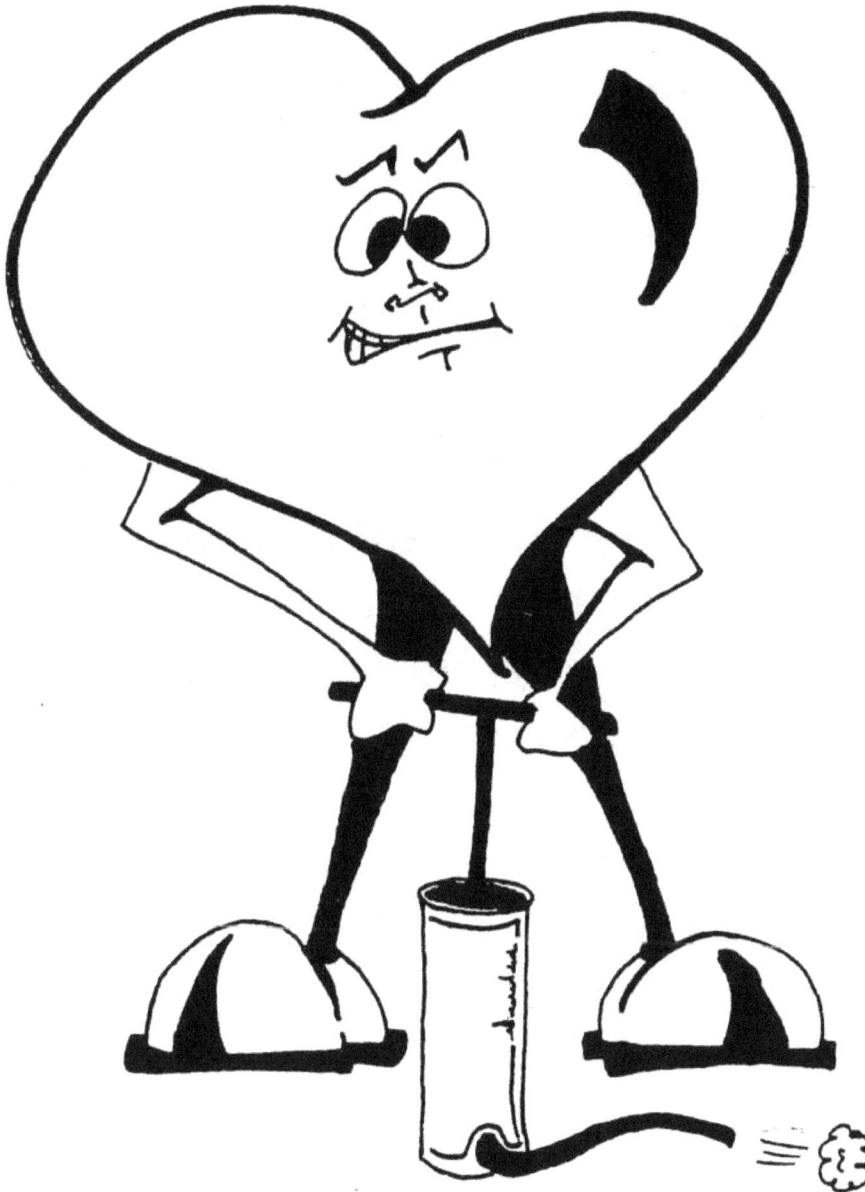

Simplified Hemodynamics

By

Malcolm Rosenberg, R.N.
And
Steven Cohn, M.D.

Hemodynamics means movement of blood. In a typical hemodynamic measurement you will see the amount of blood flowing, the
pressure to make it flow, and the resistance's to flow. These amounts,
pressures, and resistance's are measured both for the heart as a single pump
and particular areas within the heart.

During my critical care course a few years ago I dug up just about every book
on the subject. Maybe I was prejudiced, but none of them were very good.
The main problem was the pictures. They looked like a real heart.

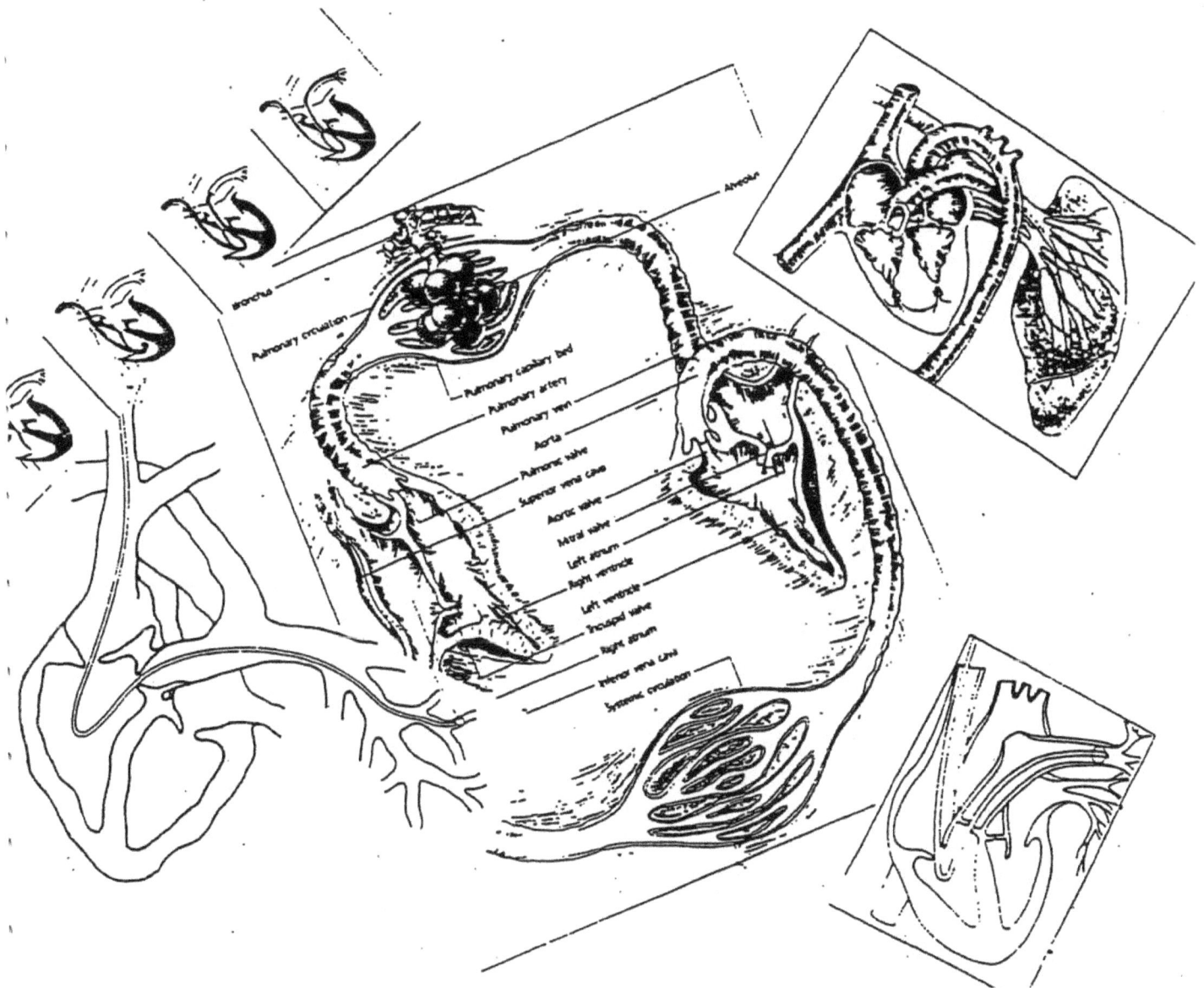

But that obscured the hemodynamics, the volumes, pressures and resistance's. Especially the huge aorta that covers everything. Tlo solve that problem, I reduced all drawings to one simple diagram. It is a plumbing schematic diagram that shows the heart as a set of pumps, pipes. and valves.

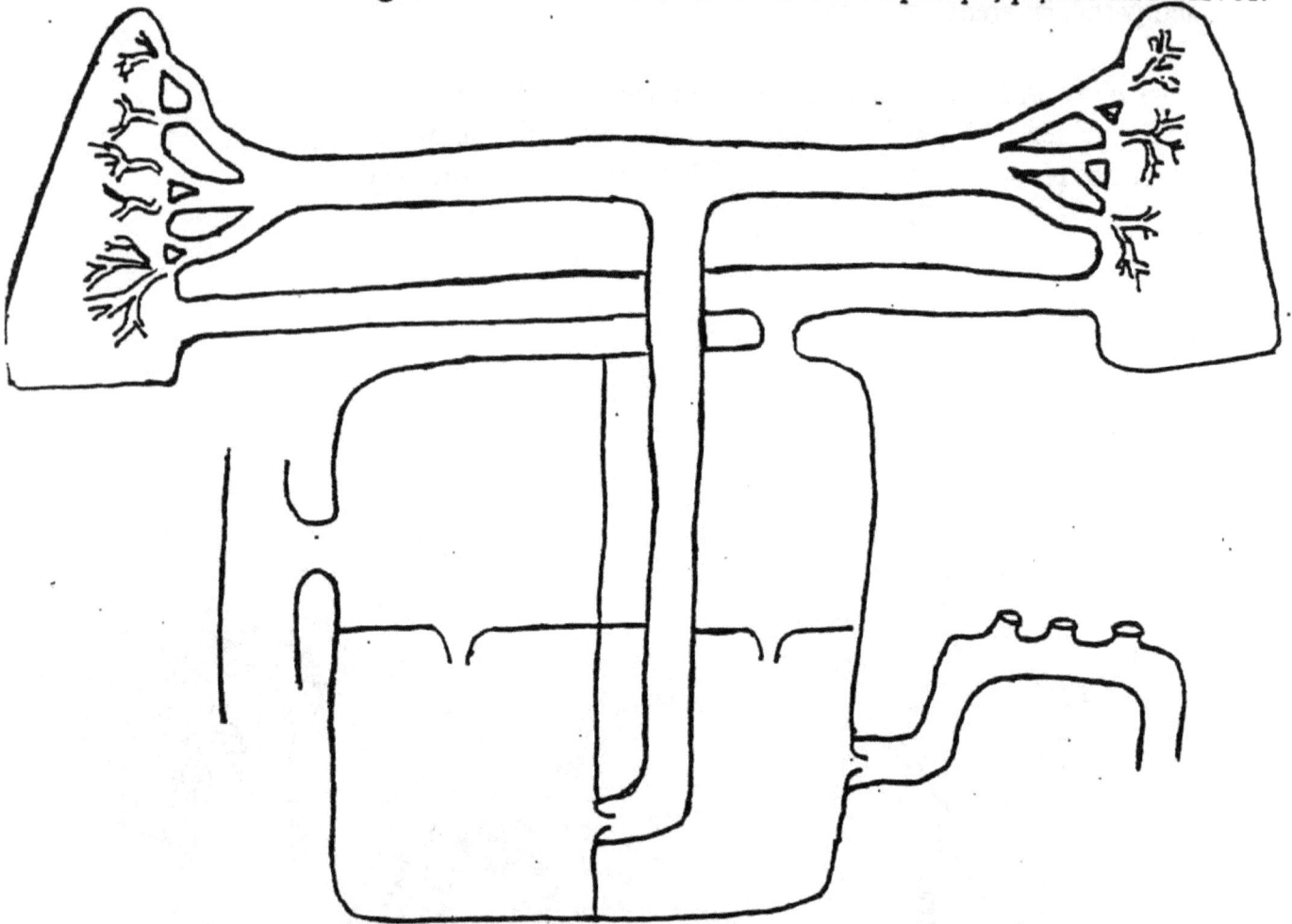

Another problem l wrestled with was the order of material.. There is no perfect sequence of arrangement. If something doesn't follow naturally, my appologies. I did the best I could. We start with hemodynamic definitions. Then we progress to the mechanics of the Swan-Ganz catheter. Finally we get into the heart's pumping action as seen through a swan.

Like my other three books, this one is very simple. If you read it, and if necessary reread it, I am sure you can learn the material. So, let's go! Turn the page.

What is a Swan-Ganz Catheter?

I'm sure you know that blood is very important. It has to get to all six trillion cells in your body. That means squeezing through millions of very, very tiny cappillaries barely larger than a single red blood cell. That is to say blood does not just swoosh around your body. Flowing through a huge pipeline like the aorta is a cinch.

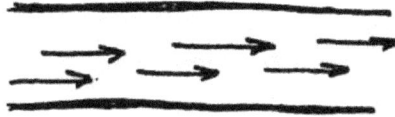

but flowing through all those cappillaries is pretty tough

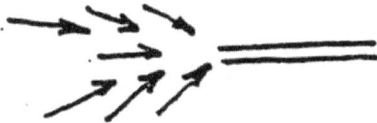

That's why we need a pump otherwise known as the heart. Unfortunately when it isn't working right we also need cardiologists. I'm sure many of you readers could think of some cardiologists you don't need. .
  When the blood doesn't flow around your body like it should, there could be many sources of the problem. To see exactly what the problem is they could use a Swan-Ganz catheter. A swan can usually pin point the exact problem in the heart or vasculature. It gives us blood pressures in different parts of the heart and the volume of blood pumped.

Now I will explain the most basic features of a swan. To avoid confusion, I am intentionally skipping a lot of material : the ports, injection sites and procedures. Right now we're just looking at its ability to tell us blood pressures. A swan is a long tube that is usually threaded from the subclavian vein through the superior vena cava into the heart.

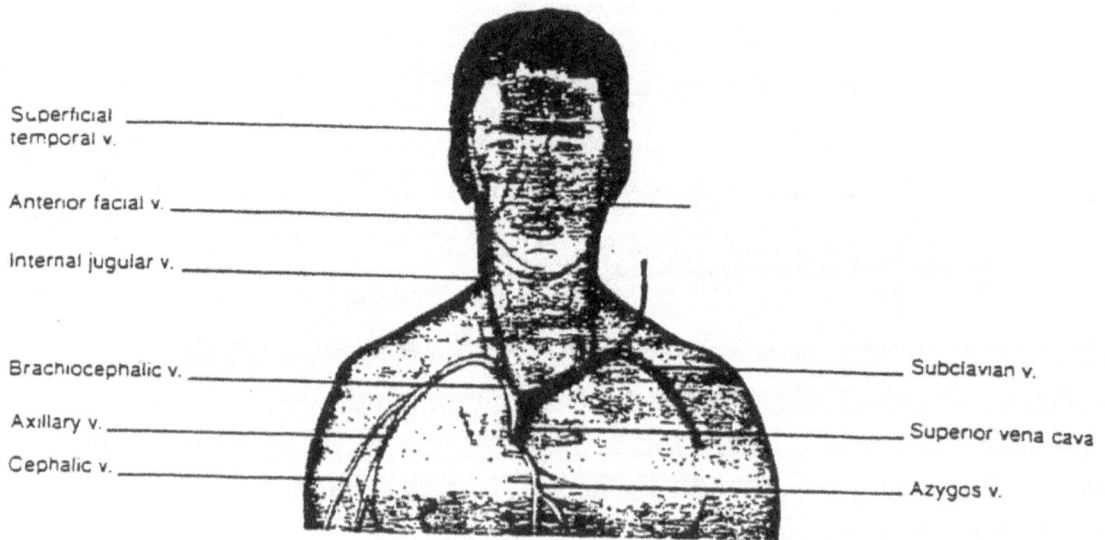

Superficial temporal v.
Anterior facial v.
Internal jugular v.
Brachiocephalic v.
Axillary v.
Cephalic v.
Subclavian v.
Superior vena cava
Azygos v.

It has a pressure sensor on the tip. The pressure shows up on a screen that gives the numerical value and a graphical picture of the pressure changes. If the pressure is changing as in a heart beat the high and low values are given (systolic and diastolic).

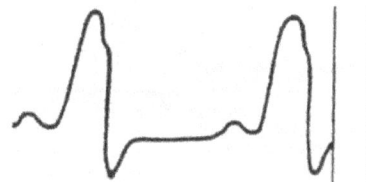

21
8

The other major feature of a swan is a 1 cc balloon near the distal tip - very much like a foley catheter. It is inflated with a 1 cc syringe very much like a foley catheter. When the catheter is inflated and the balloon gets stuck in a branch of the pulmonary artery its called a "wedge". I will go into much, much more detail on this later. But very briefly the wedged catheter tip occludes any blood flow from behind it.

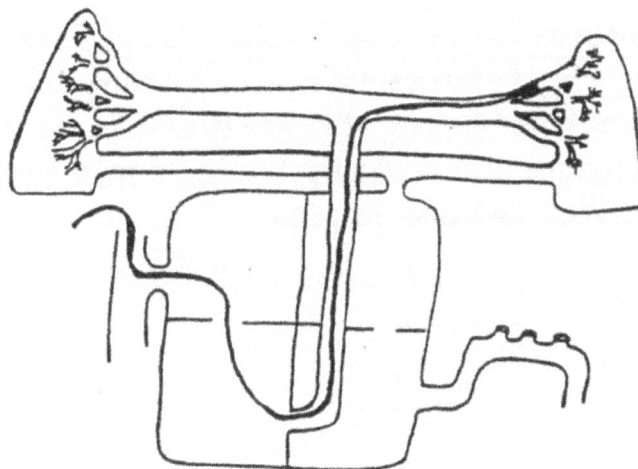

The pressure sensor on the tip measures only the blood pressure distal to it. Thats a Swan-Ganz in a nut shell. The next 50 pages explain it in more detail.

SOME HEMODYNAMIC DEFINITIONS

Turn the page.

SOME HEMODYNAMIC DEFINITIONS

Arterial Blood Pressure

You probably are quite familiar with blood pressure. This is certainly the most frequently used hemodynamic measurement. Let's look at it a little more closely.

When a fluid (like blood) flows freely through a large tube (like your arteries), it is called **laminar flow**. It is very smooth and doesn't make any noise.

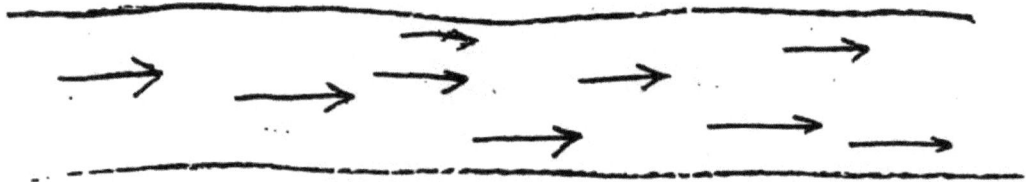

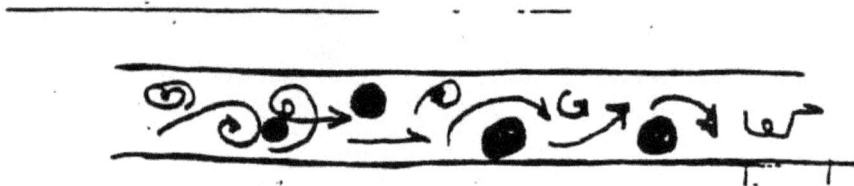

When there are obstructions to the flow we call it turbulent. Turbulent is noisy. You've seen this: a quietly flowing stream that has to gush its way around some big rocks. It's much noisier. Pertaining to our arteries, turbulent flow is also created by a narrowing of the channel.

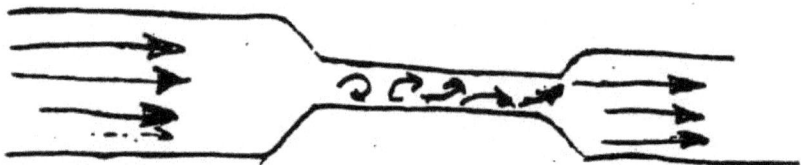

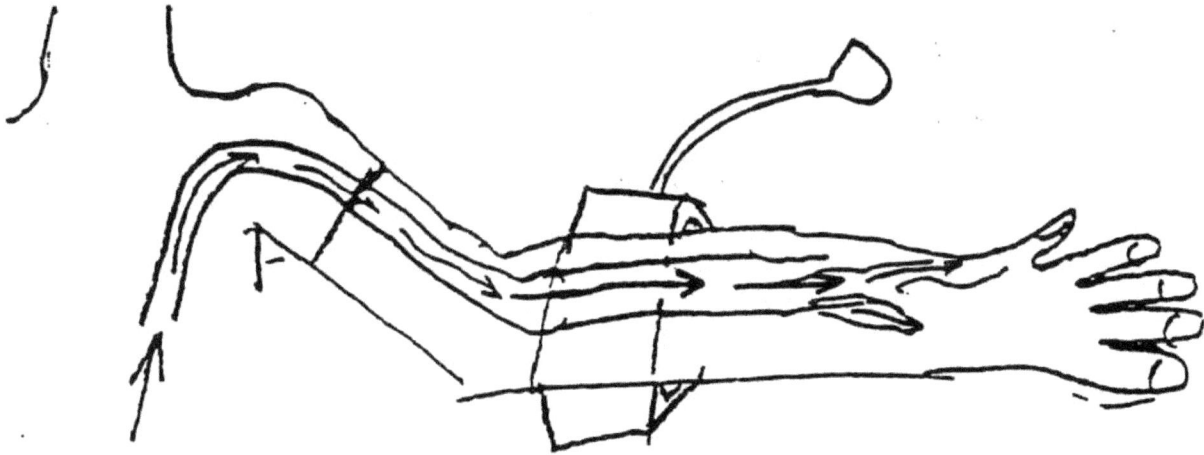

We measure blood pressure with a blood pressure cuff - a sphygmomanometer. Putting your stethoscope on the artery you hear nothing because the flow is smooth, unobstructed.

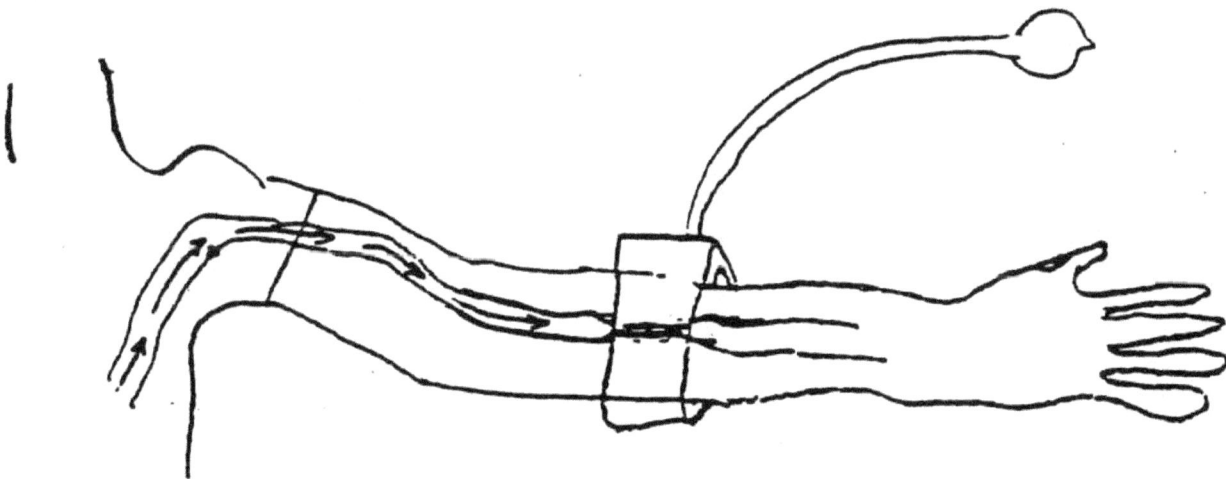

Then you inflate the cuff to completely clamp off blood flow.

When you start to hear thumping that's systolic blood pressure. The amount of pressure to overcome the pumping action of the heart. Completely stopping the flow so you hear nothing.

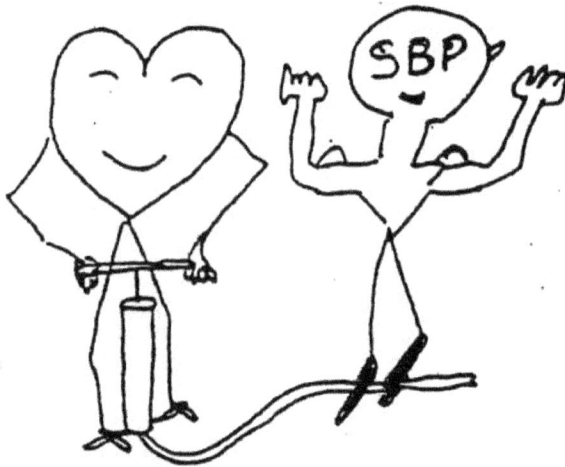

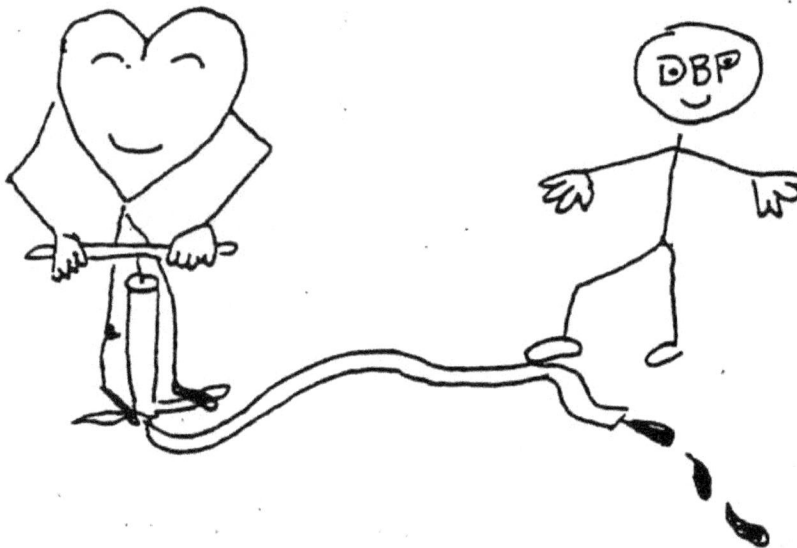

Diastolic blood pressure is how much pressure is exerted to open the arteries sufficiently to allow free flow of blood – and no noise.

In between completely plugged and totally free flow you hear the thumping – the turbulent flow.

Cardiac Output

Cardiac output is the amount of blood that the heart pumps per minute

Normal values are 4 to 15 liters. That's a lot, 1 to 4 gallons. Cardiac output is the amount of blood pumped each minute. About 5 liters or 5 quarts is normal. An olympic athelete could pump up to 35 liters a minute during a race.

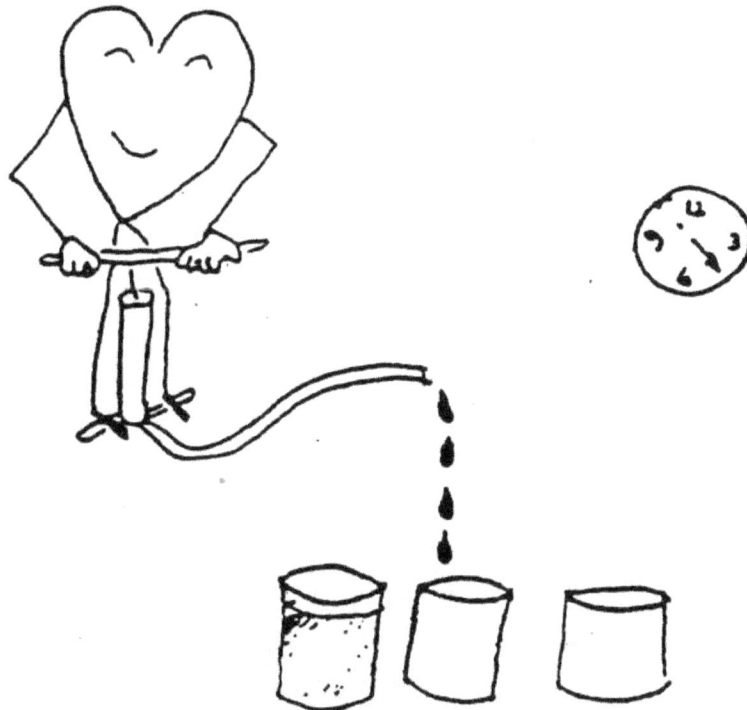

Cardiac Index

The cardiac output gives a good idea of the heart's output. But it does not give any indication about the body's need for blood.

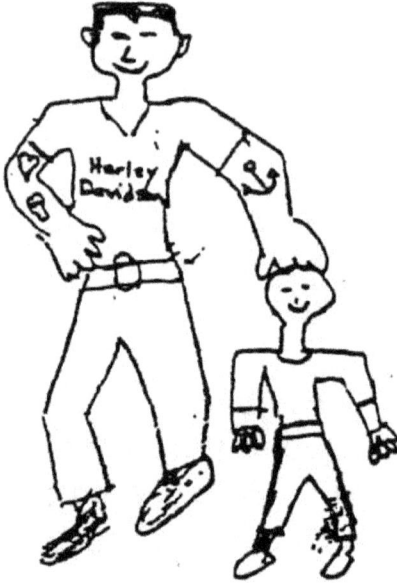

This guy's body obviously requires more blood than this guy. To get the cardiac index divide the cardiac output by the body surface area. Body surface area can be calculated from a chart. All you need is the height and weight.

Step # 1: Get the height and weight.

Step # 2: Get the body surface area from a chart using the height and weight (see example)

Step # 3: Divide cardiac output by body surface area.

Body Surface of Adults

Nomogram for determination of body surface from height and mass'

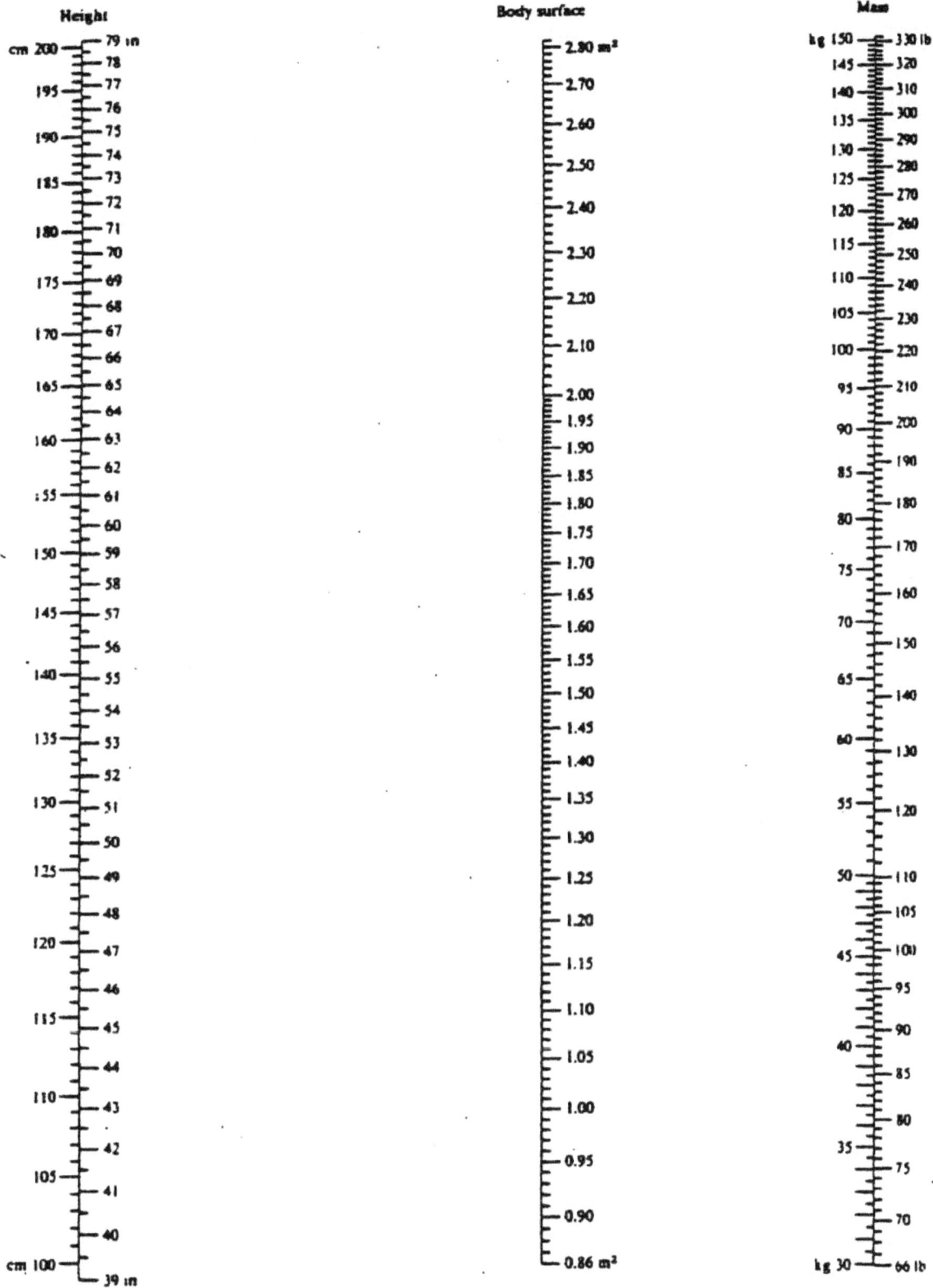

Height	Body surface	Mass

Height

cm 200 — 79 in
78
195 — 77
76
190 — 75
74
185 — 73
72
180 — 71
70
175 — 69
68
170 — 67
66
165 — 65
64
160 — 63
62
155 — 61
60
150 — 59
58
145 — 57
56
140 — 55
54
135 — 53
52
130 — 51
50
125 — 49
48
120 — 47
46
115 — 45
44
110 — 43
42
105 — 41
40
cm 100 — 39 in

Body surface

2.80 m²
2.70
2.60
2.50
2.40
2.30
2.20
2.10
2.00
1.95
1.90
1.85
1.80
1.75
1.70
1.65
1.60
1.55
1.50
1.45
1.40
1.35
1.30
1.25
1.20
1.15
1.10
1.05
1.00
0.95
0.90
0.86 m²

Mass

kg 150 — 330 lb
145 — 320
140 — 310
135 — 300
130 — 290
125 — 280
270
120 — 260
115 — 250
110 — 240
105 — 230
100 — 220
95 — 210
90 — 200
85 — 190
180
80 — 170
75 — 160
70 — 150
65 — 140
60 — 130
55 — 120
50 — 110
105
101
45 — 95
90
40 — 85
80
35 — 75
70
kg 30 — 66 lb

Values are method dependent.

From Lentner C. Geigy scientific tables, 8ed. Basel: Ciba-Geigy Ltd.

Stroke Volume

Stroke volume is the amount of blood squirted with each heartbeat. So naturally you divide the cardiac output (the volume pumped in a minute) by the heart rate, the number of beats per minute to get the stroke volume.

Mean Arterial Pressure

Mean arterial pressure is kind of like the average pressure in your arteries. The formula is:

Mean Arterial Pressure = $\dfrac{2x \text{ diastolic BP} + \text{Systolic BP}}{3}$

It multiples the diastolic by two because diastolic last longer then systolic.

Systemic Vascular Resistance

   We measure just how tough it is by systemic vascular resistance. To calculate SVR the formula is $\underline{(MAP-CVP) \times 80}$.
                    CO

I won't try to make sense of that formula. But you can sort of get the gist of it. The Mean Arterial Pressure is pressure in the arteries or the blood pressure right after the blood has left the heart. The Central Venous pressure is the pressure right before it gets back to the heart. Kind of like the pressure drop in the garden hose.

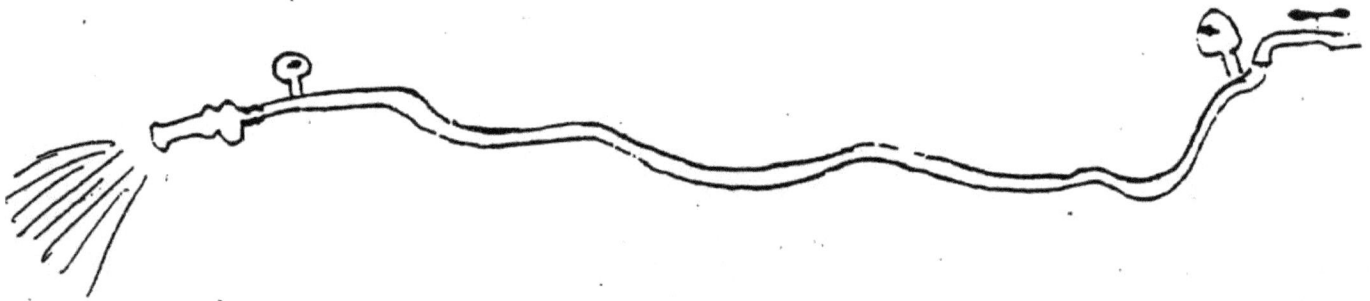

   You divide that pressure drop by how much blood is flowing - the cardiac output. If a lot of blood is flowing than you are dividing by a bigger number which means a smaller systemic vascular resistance. And that sort of makes sense - more blood flow implies less resistance.

   Another way to look at it is:

Blood flow = $\underline{pressure}$ or   resistance = $\dfrac{pressure}{blood\ flow}$
                resistance

   Just don't forget the "80."

The Swan-Ganz catheter was designed by two doctors, Dr. Harold "Hairy Bird" Swan and Dr. William "Wild Bill" Ganz.

A Swan-Ganz catheter is used to measure pressures in different parts of the heart and lungs. The pressures usually show on a screen with the number and a graphic picture of the pressures.

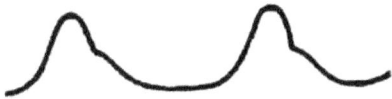

The "**swan,**" as you'll soon be calling it, is inserted through the right side of the heart. The insertion is similar to a central line - usually into the subclavian vein or left internal jugular vein.

From there it passes through the superior vena cava. The pressure here is called central venous pressure. Normal values are 0-5mmHg.

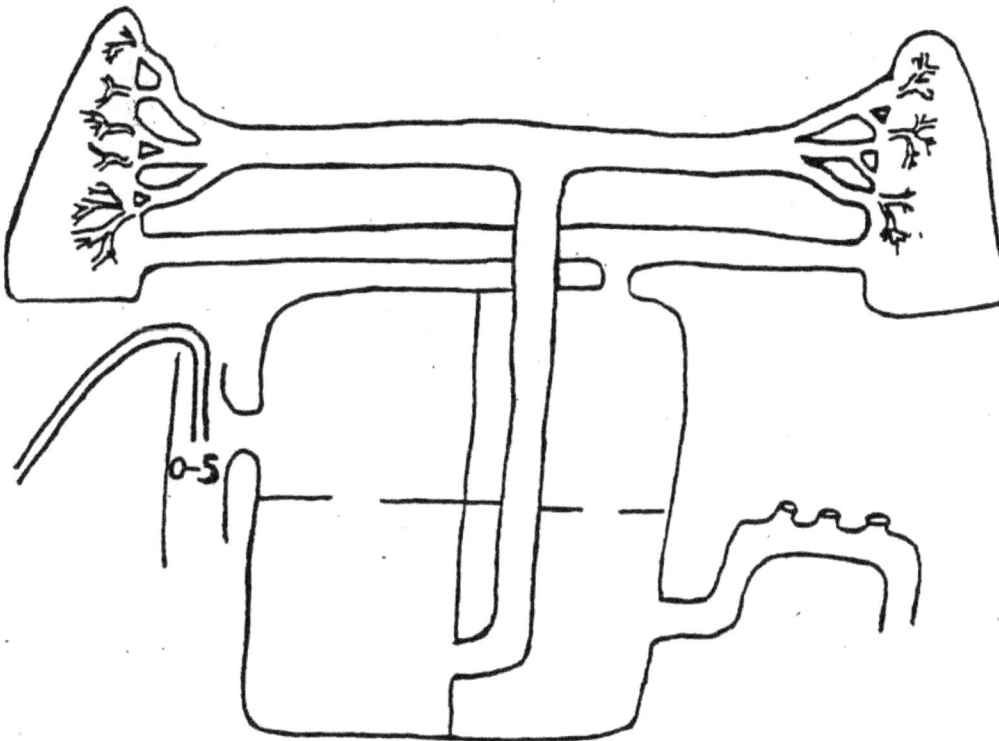

Next, as the doctor continues to advance the catheter, you will see the smooth line start to vary. This indicates the tip is in the right atrium. You would expect this since the atria do have small pumping actions. So it shows as small waves. Normal values are 2-5mmHg. At this point the balloon is inflated. This enables the catheter tip to "go with the flow." The blood flow pulls the catheter tip through the tricuspid valve.

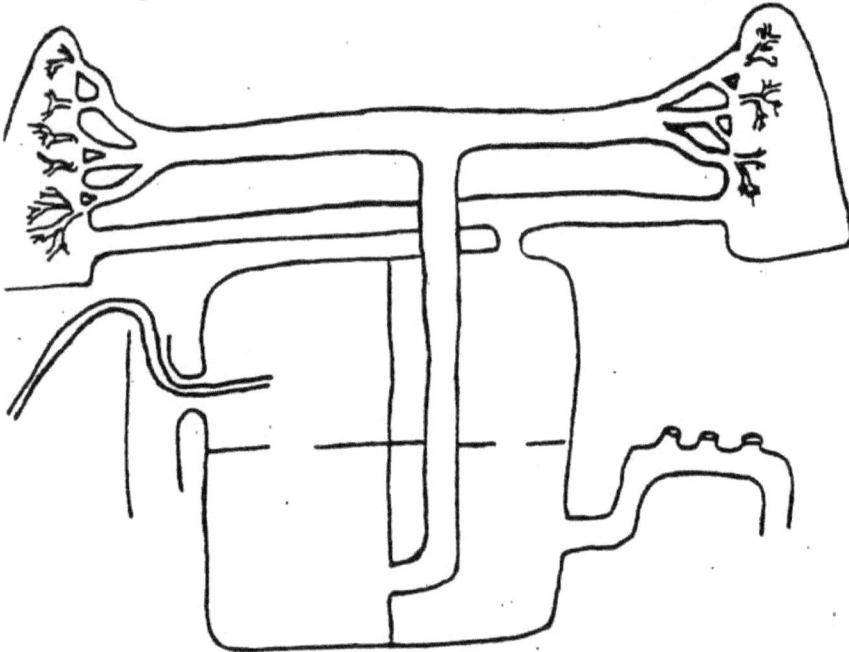

The tip continues and passes through the tricuspid valve into the right ventricle. Again, you know it's position by changes in the pressure wave form. You can clearly see the ventricle contracting by the systolic and diastolic pressures. Normal values are 20/2.

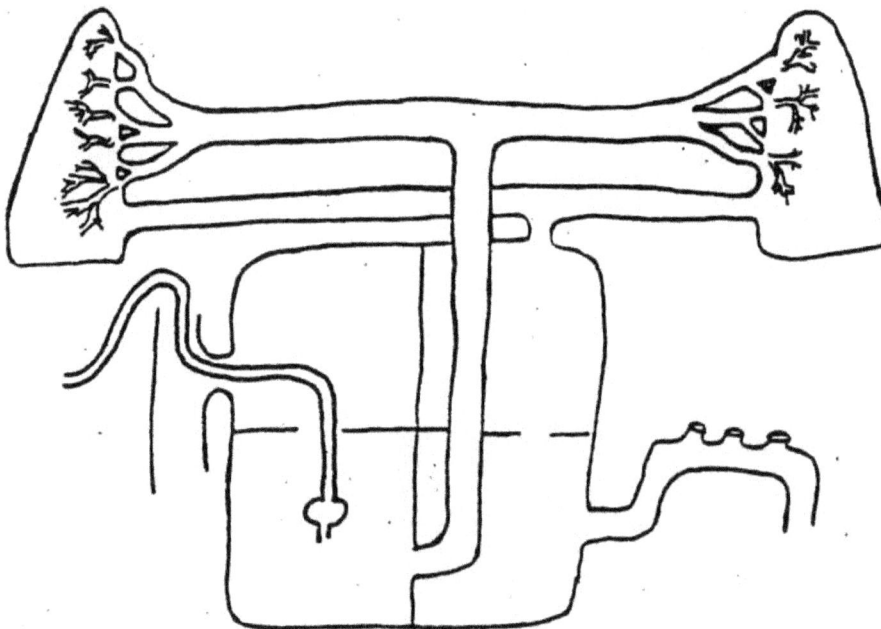

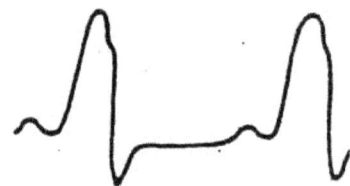

The tip must continue to flow past the right ventricle. You wouldn't want the probe to hang around too long in the right ventricle. Your heart's reaction to a lingering probe is sort of the way you feel about a sigmoidoscopy. You'd throw lots of PVC's- to say the least.

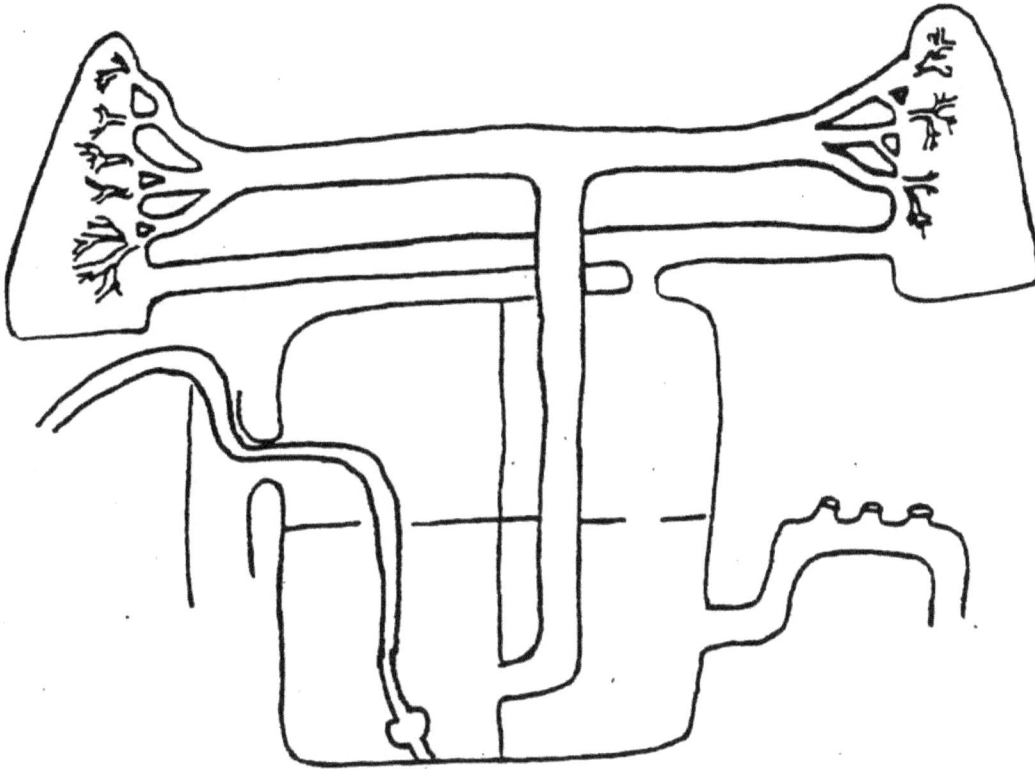

Ouch!

The probe leaves the ventricle, passes through the pulmonic valve and enters the pulmonary artery. Again, we know where the probe is by the wave form. The wave form is clearly arterial. By "**arterial**," we mean *formed by the pumping action and the valves opening and closing*. This same form would appear when taking blood pressures with an "A" line in the radial artery.

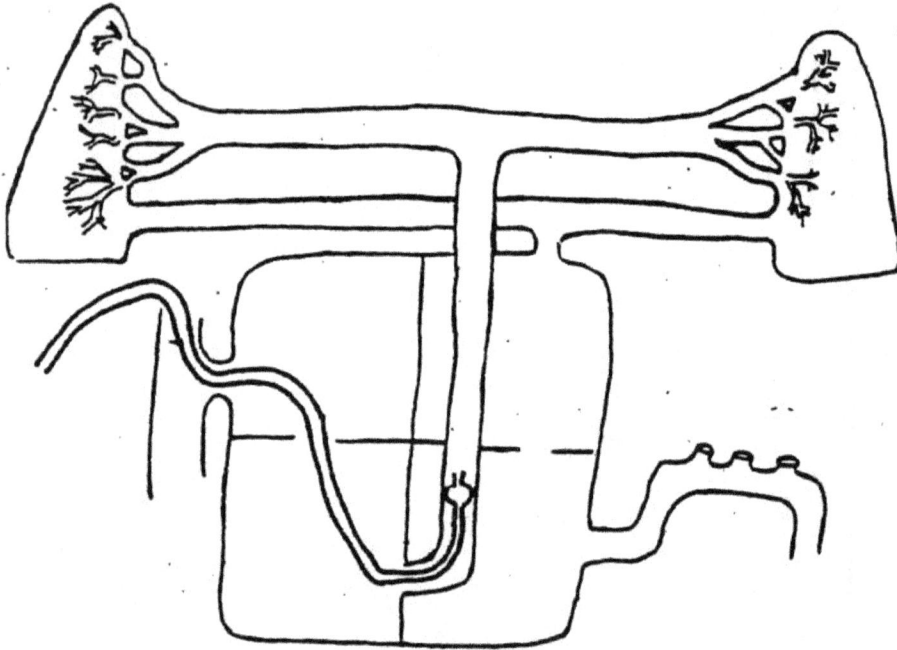

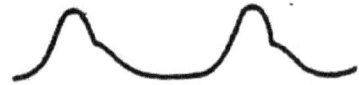

Let's look more closely at the arterial wave form. Remember the probe is in the pulmonary artery. First, the ventricle contracts. Blood gushes into the artery and pressure rises. This is seen as a sharp rise in pressure. The peak is the systolic blood pressure.

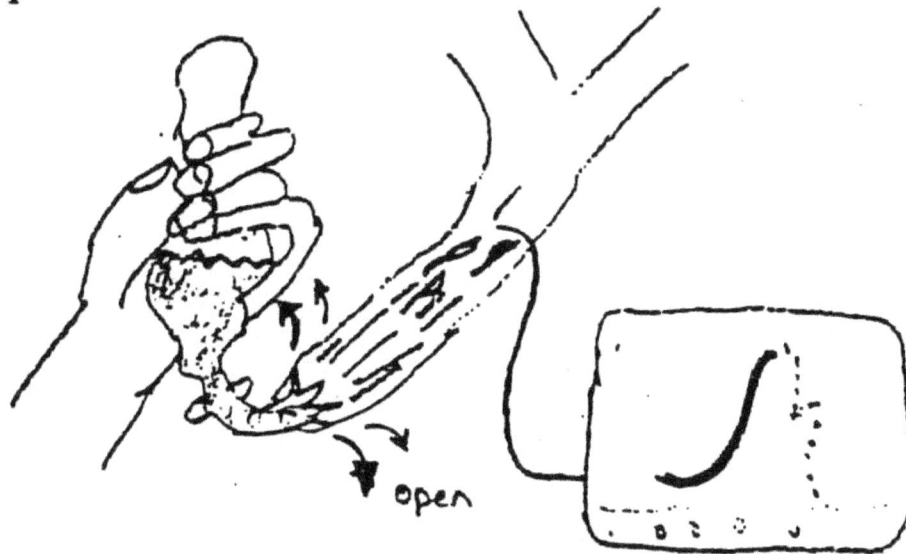

After almost all of the blood is squeezed out, the volume of blood spurting falls. We see this on the screen.

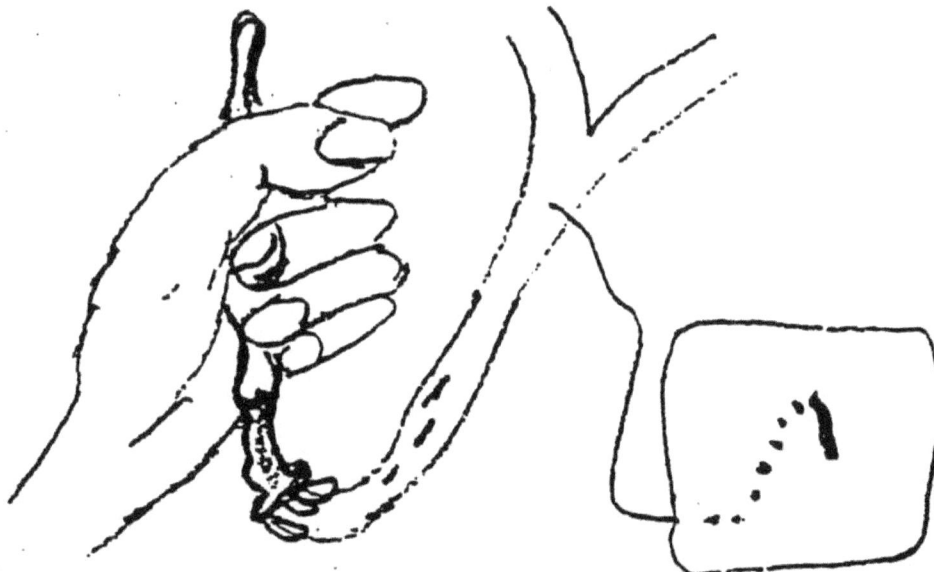

When there is no more blood, the pulmonic valve snaps shut, you'll see a short, flat line. No more blood pushing through means no changes in pressure. That's why the line is flat. That part of the curve is called the dicrotic notch. (Sometimes it is mistakenly called the necrotic crotch.) The pressure continues to fall as the remaining blood continues to flow into the pulmonary artery and lungs.

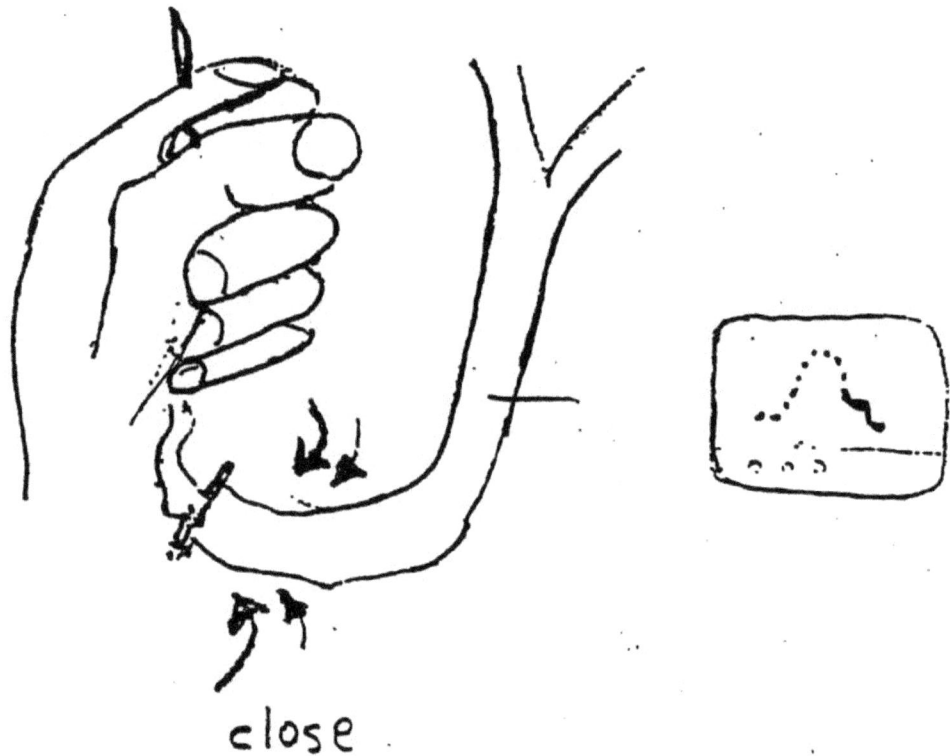

close

WEDGE PRESSURE

We said the probe has reached the pulmonary artery. In fact it has reached into one of the two branches. At this point we can get the wedge pressure (or wedgie). What we're trying to do is look into the left atrium without being there.

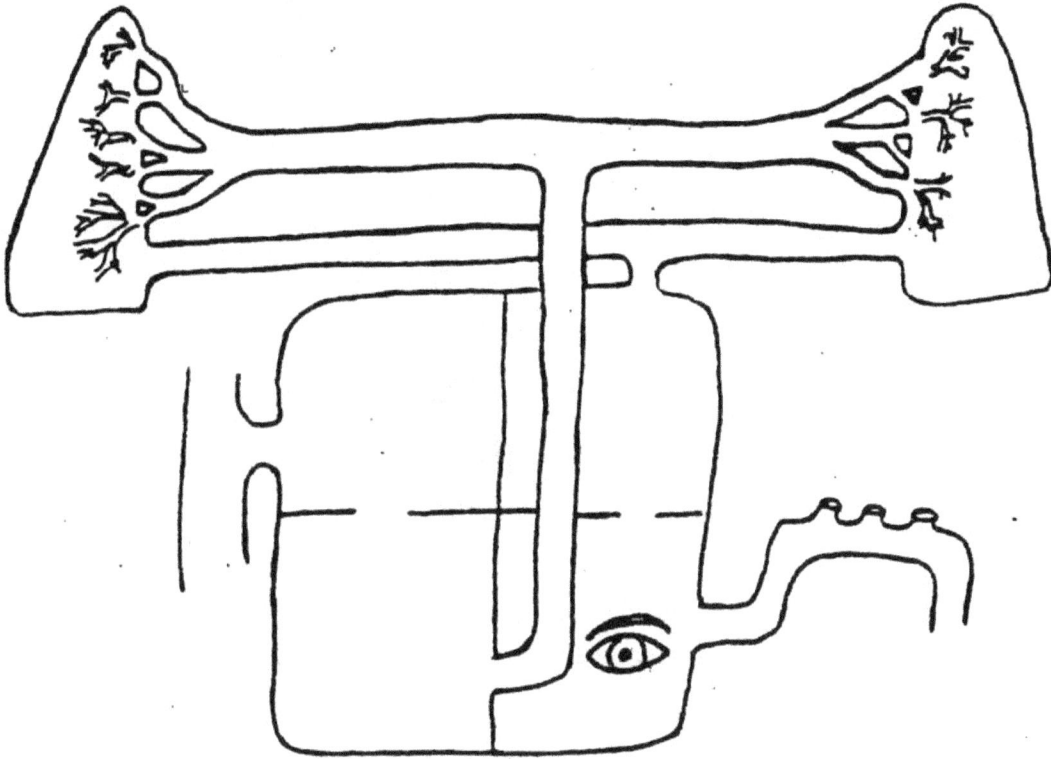

Most cardiac action is in the left ventricle. There are plenty of other things that can go wrong (ask any cardiologist). For the most part, good left ventricular pumping means adequate perfusion. How do we look into the left atrium without being there?

Let's review cardiac pumping. Oxygenated blood returns to the left atrium from the lungs through the pulmonary vein. The atrium fills while the left ventricle is contracting (systole). The pressure from the squeezed blood forces the mitral valve flaps closed.

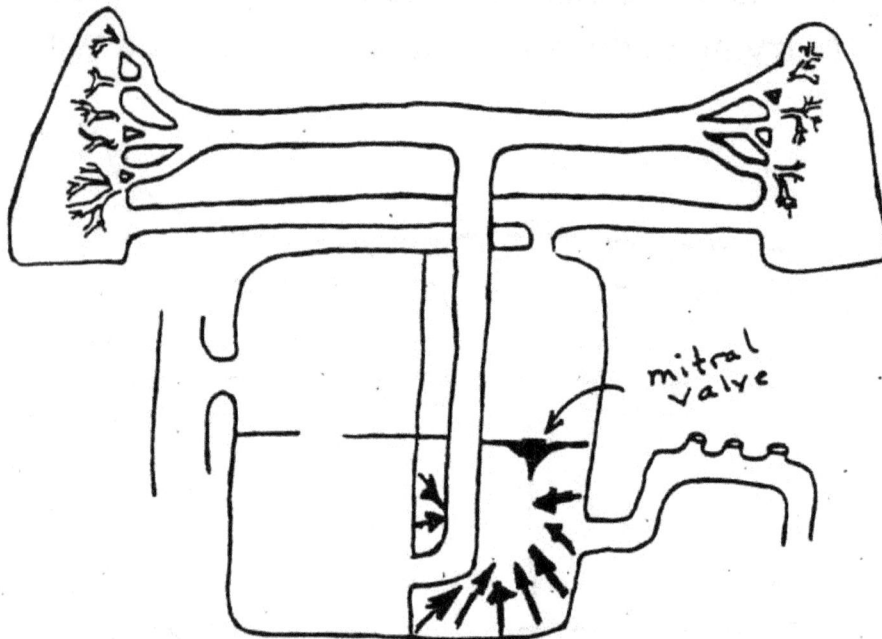

mitral valve

The ventricle finishes its contraction. It has squeezed out all the blood that's gonna get squeezed. That's called the ejection fraction, normally about 60%.

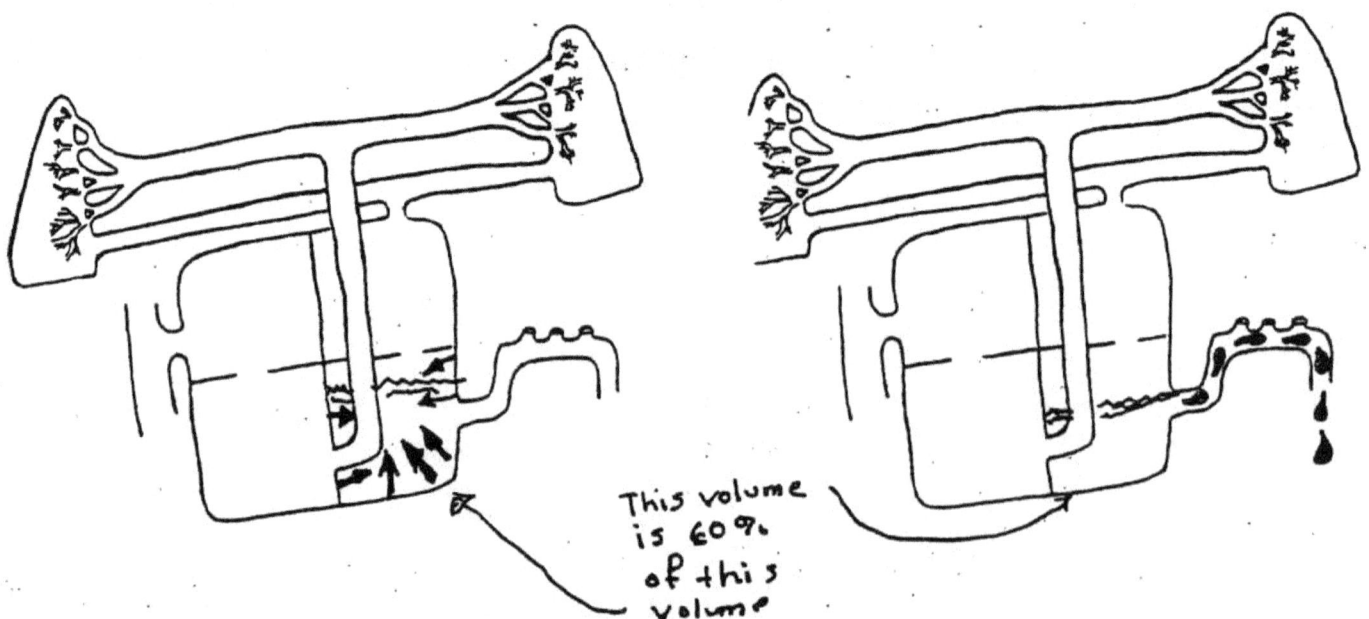

This volume is 60% of this volume

After the ventricle relaxes (in ventricular diastole), the flaps on the mitral valve fall open.

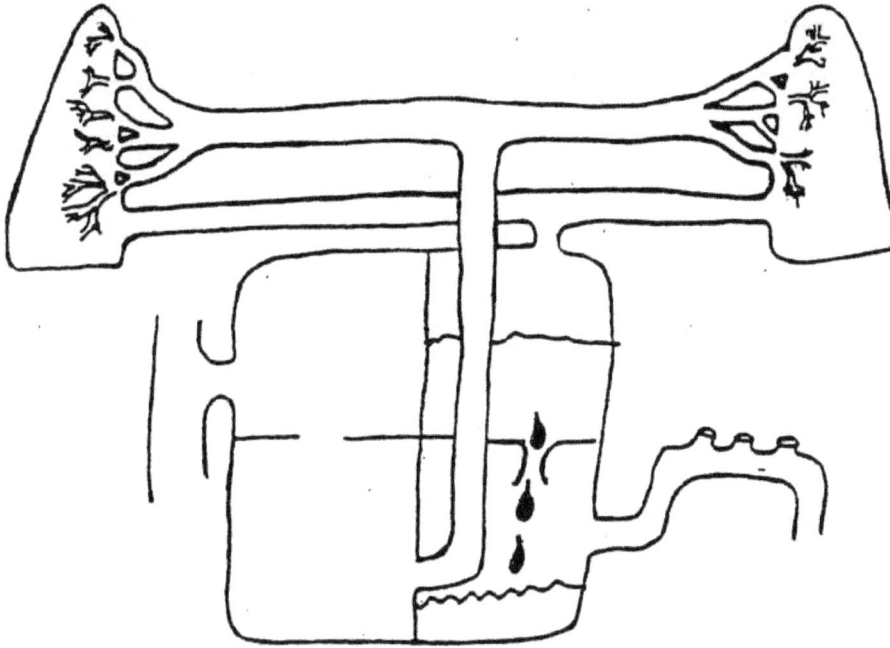

The atria drops about 75% of the blood then squeezes out the rest. That's atrial systole which happens at the same time as ventricular diastole. At the end of the atrial squeeze is **ventricular end diastole.** In the left ventricle, which we are talking about now, it's **left ventricular end diastole.** The pressure in the left ventricle at the end of diastole is **left ventricular end diastolic pressure.** Like all other blood pressures, it is in millimeters of mercury (mmHg).

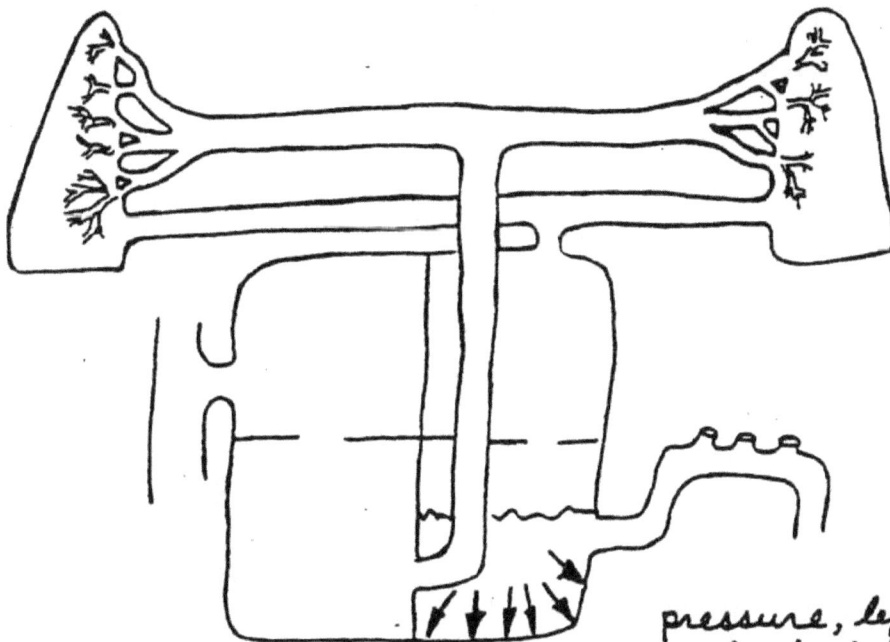

pressure, left ventricular end diastolic pressure

Filling the ventricle, just like this balloon, stretches the walls. That's called preload, the pressure of the blood in the ventricle just sitting there caused by the stretching of the walls. The blood left from the last contraction, plus what the atrium has just squeezed in, stretches the walls to produce **LVEDP**.

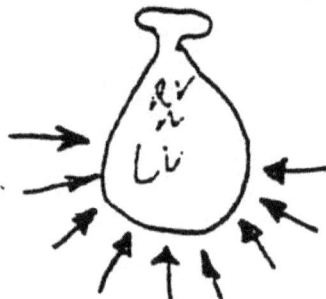

The left ventricular diastolic pressure is very revealing about left ventricular function. That one pressure tells us alot about how the left ventricle is functioning.

You recall the **ejection fraction** is the fraction of the blood squeezed out of the ventricle with each heart beat. A 50% ejection fraction means that 50% of the blood is squeezed out in each contraction..

How does that relate to pressure? **LVEDP** to be exact? Simple: If the ventricle were empty prior to it's contraction, there would be no pressure. Look at this balloon.

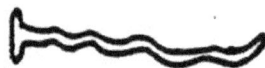

A less efficient ventricular contraction obviously leaves more blood throughout diastole and especially at the end when the atrium has finished pumping. In other words, a higher **left ventricular end diastolic pressure**. Normal values are 12 to 15 mmHg.

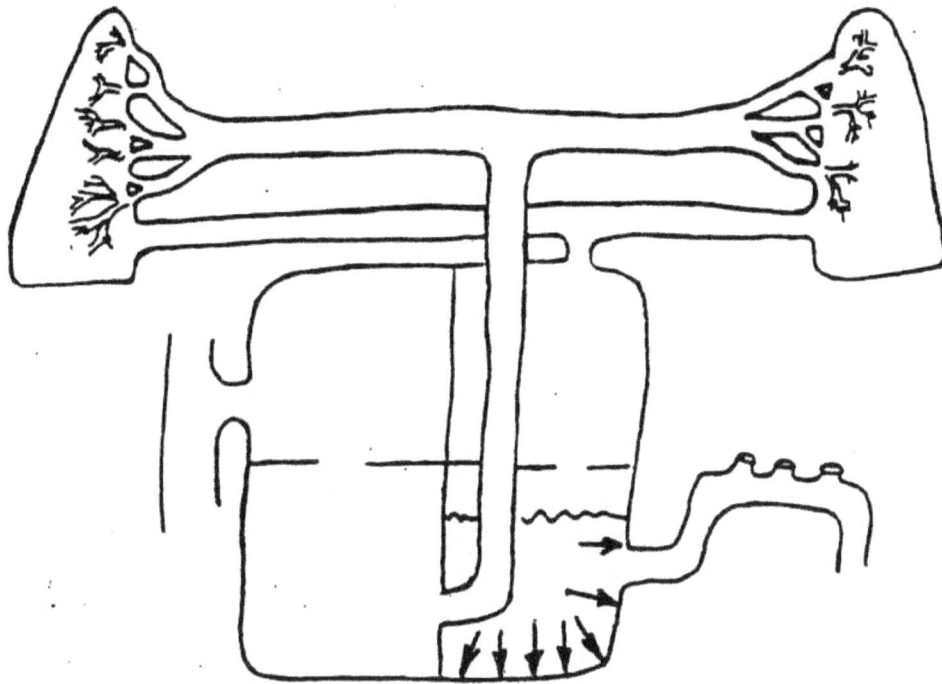

We can measure **LVEDP** 's with Swan. Here's how: The tip of the Swan-Ganz catheter is in the pulmonary artery. We blow up the balloon just like a foley catheter - with a 1 cc syringe.

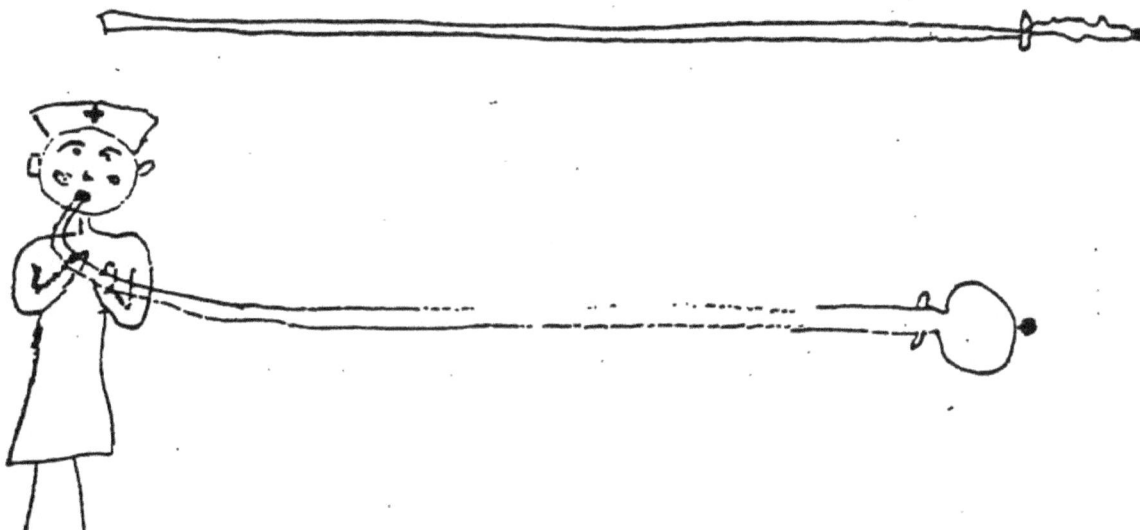

At this point I'll illustrate what the inflated does as it continues to advance. You'll notice the pumonary artery braches into smaller branches. The inflated balloon floats into progressively smaller branches until it "wedges". If the balloon is properly positioned the inflated balloon would just obstruct the branch of the pulmonary artery it is in.

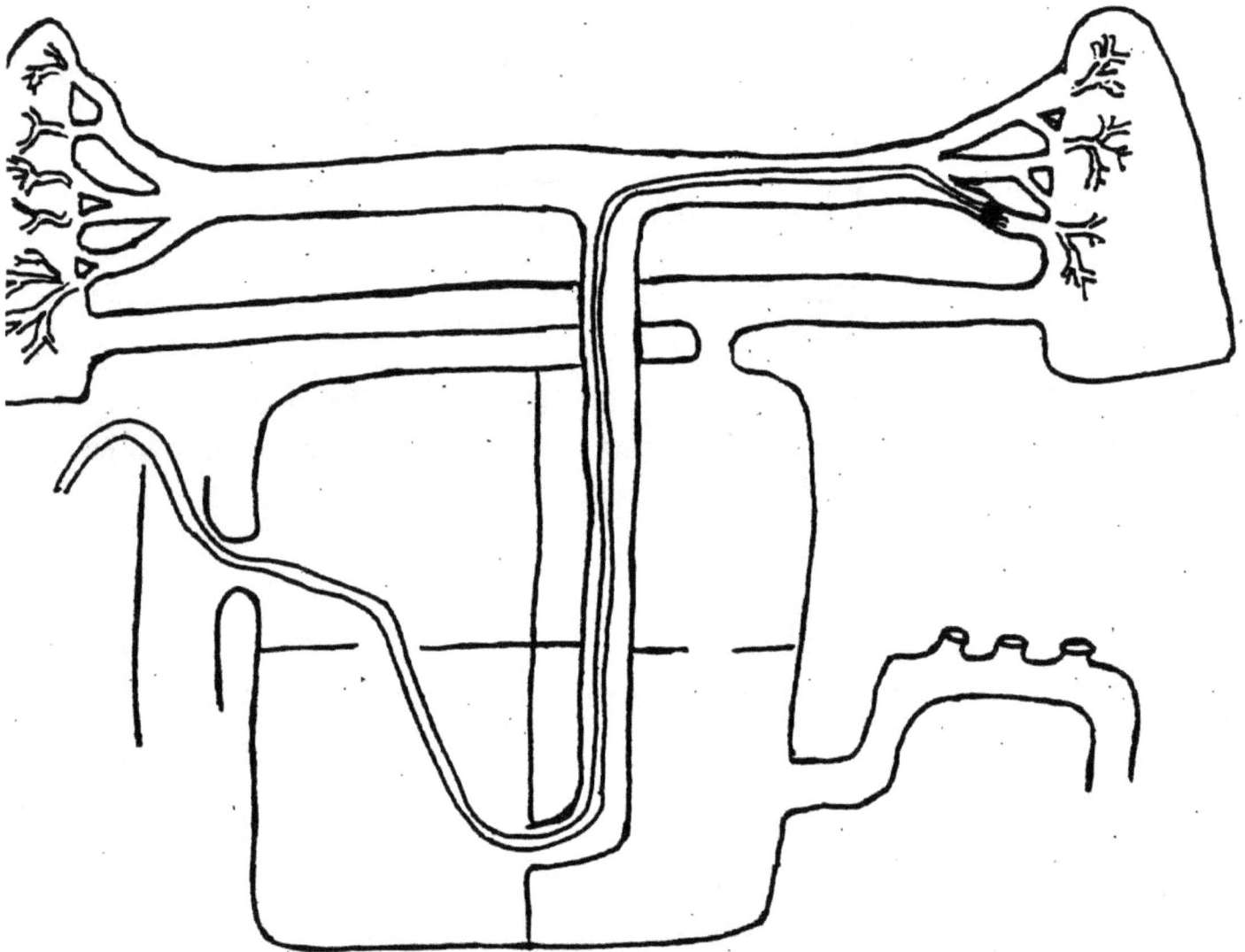

This blocks any pressure coming from the right ventricle. Notice the path from the pulmonary artery through the lungs is fairly unobstructed. That means that the tip is measuring pressure coming from the left atrium that is transmitted via the pulmonary vasculature.

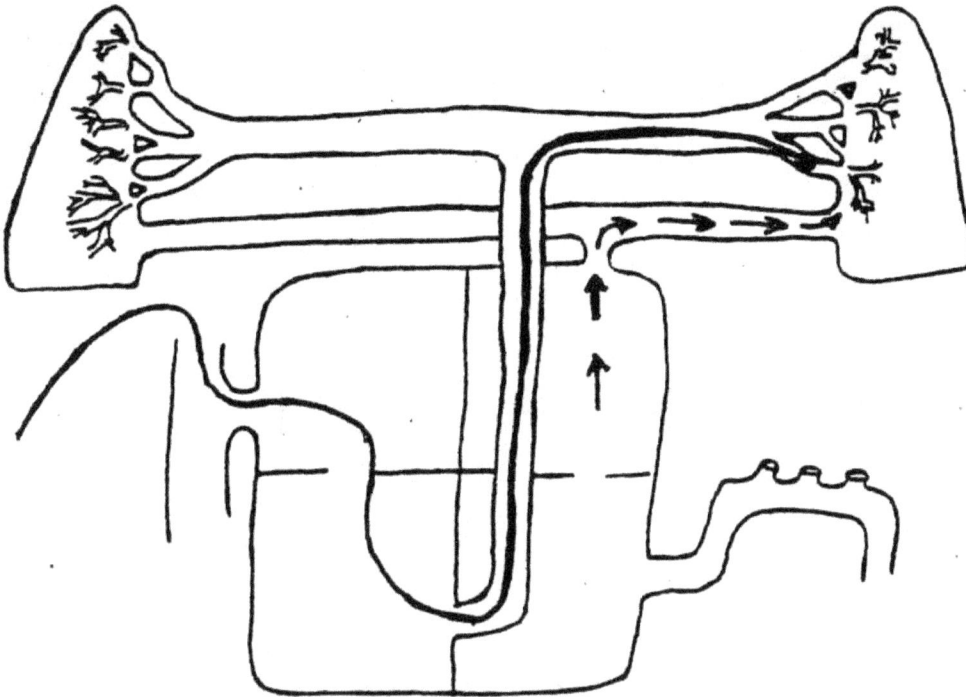

How does the pressure in the left atrium tell us anything about the left ventricle? The pressure in the left atrium is equal to the pressure in the left ventricle when the mitral valve is open.

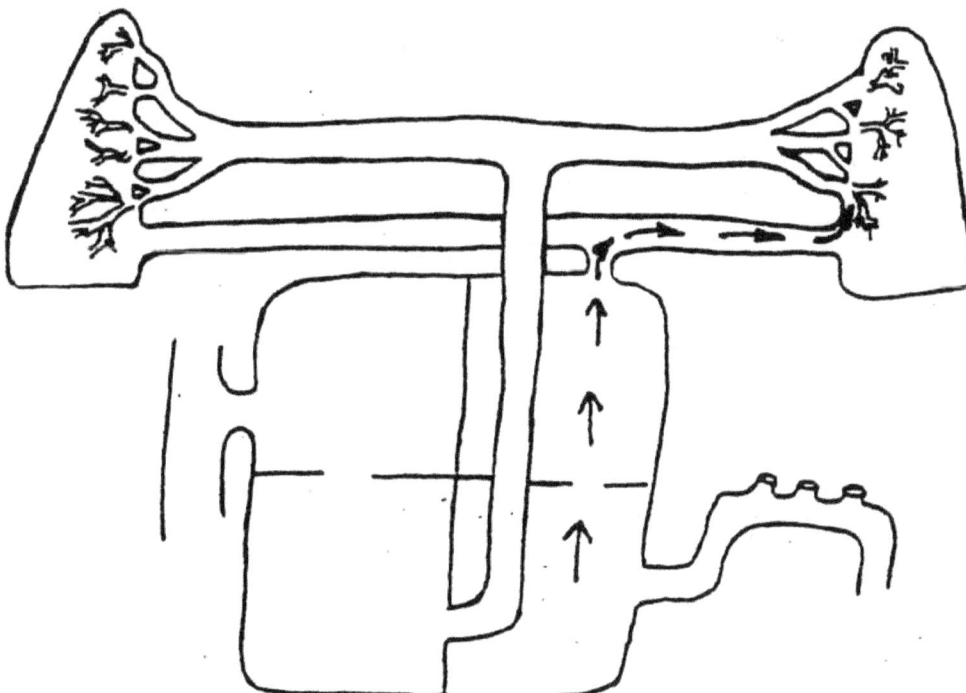

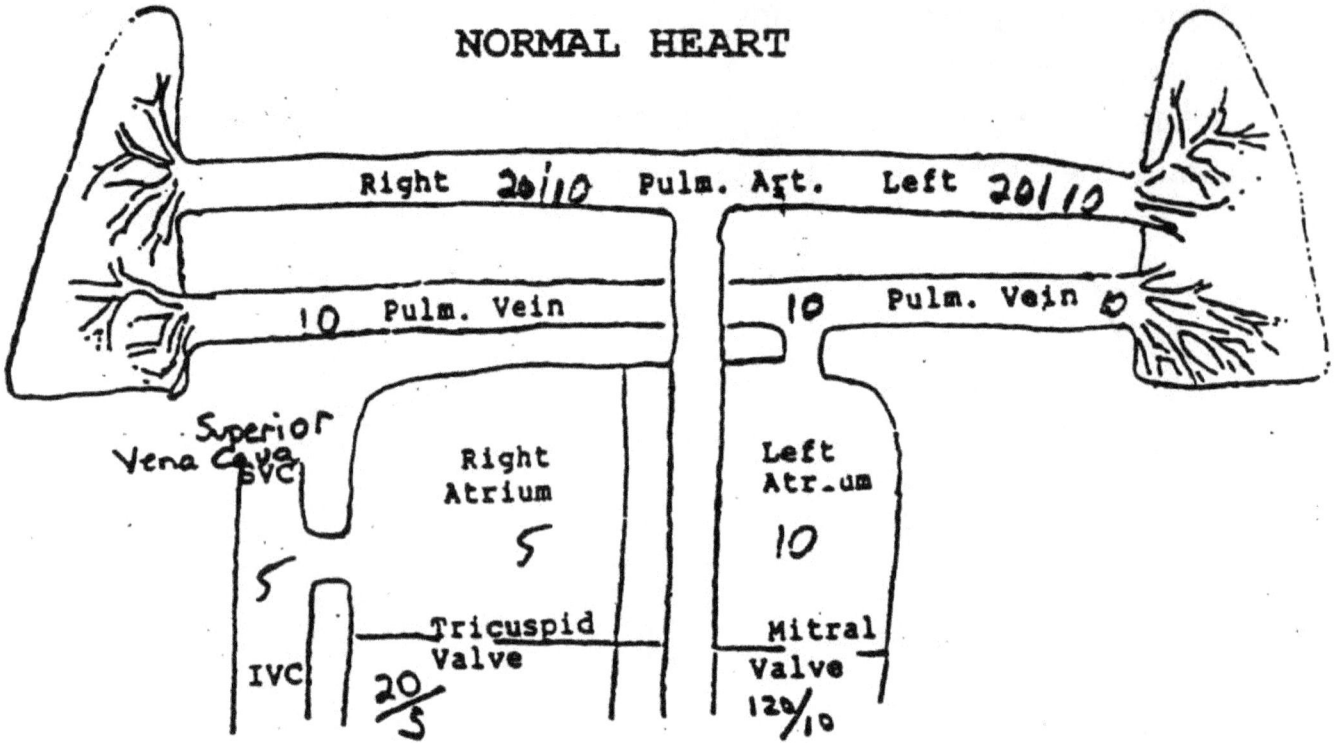

The superior vena cava supplies blood to the heart from the head and arms. The inferior vena cava supplies blood from the abdomen and legs. The pressure is very low, about 5mm Hg (venous pressure).

The blood enters the right atrium during ventricular systolic, while the tricuspid valve is closed.

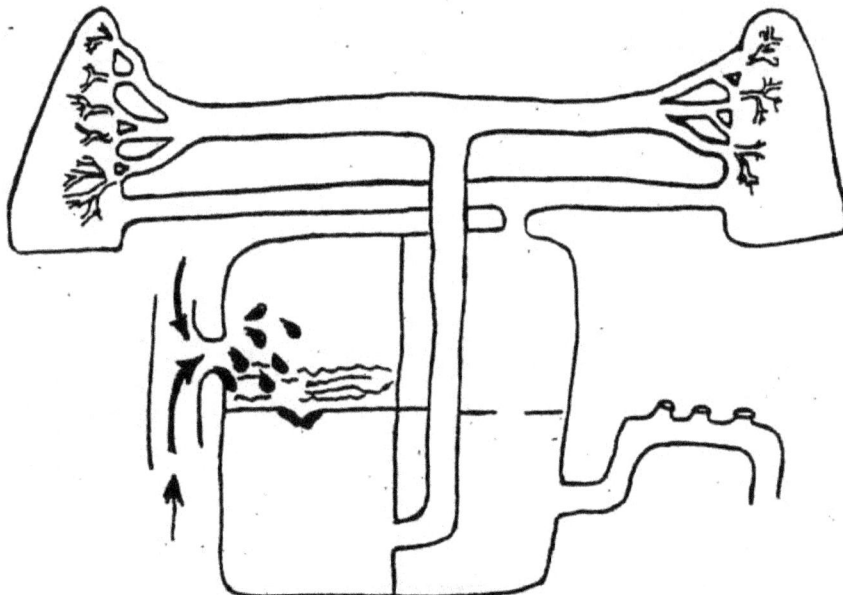

When the ventricle is relaxed, its pressure is lower than the atrium and the tricuspid valve opens. The blood just drops into the ventricle. At the end of arterial systole, it squeezes out the last 25% of blood. Notice ventricular diastolic is the same as arterial pressure.

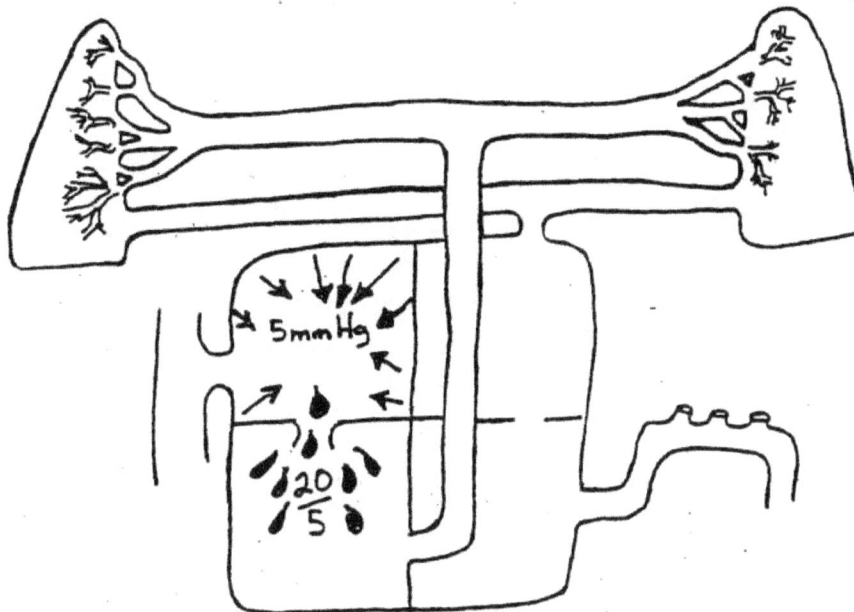

Then the ventricle starts to contract and the tricuspid valve closes. It pushes blood through the pulmonary valve into the pulmonary artery at about 20mm Hg. Notice the pulmonic artery systolic pressure is the same as the right ventricular systolic pressure.

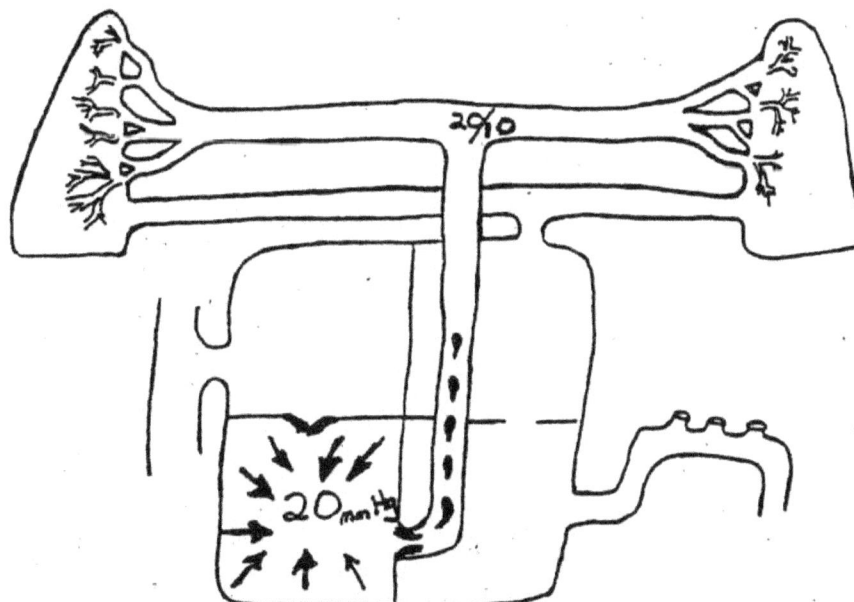

When the blood has passed from the pulmonary artery and squeezed through the small capillaries in the lungs the pressure drops. By the time it gets to the pulmonary veins the pressure is low again. Also, it is not arterial with a systolic and diastolic component any longer.

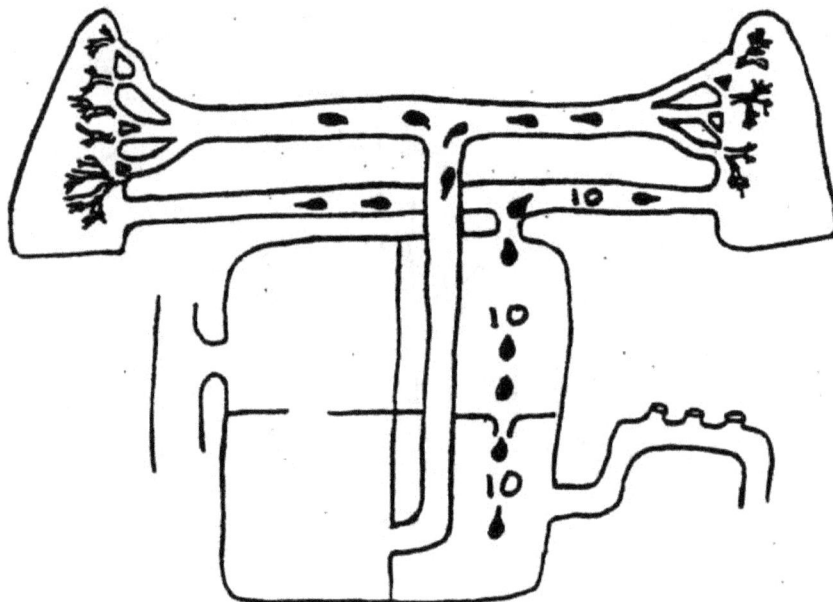

Then the whole process begins again on the left side of the heart. The left arterial pressure rises slightly as the left atrium fills. At the end of the left ventricular systole, the ventricle relaxes, the mitial valve opens, and the atria empties its contents, and the left atrium contracts. At that point we call the pressure at the left ventricle, "Left ventricular End Diastolic Pressure (LVEDP)," that is after the left atrium contracts and prior to left ventricular systole.

The left ventricle contracts vigorously and pumps blood under high pressure of about 120mm Hg. The volume of the left ventricle is about 200cc. With an ejection fraction of about 60%, 120cc are squeezed out each beat.

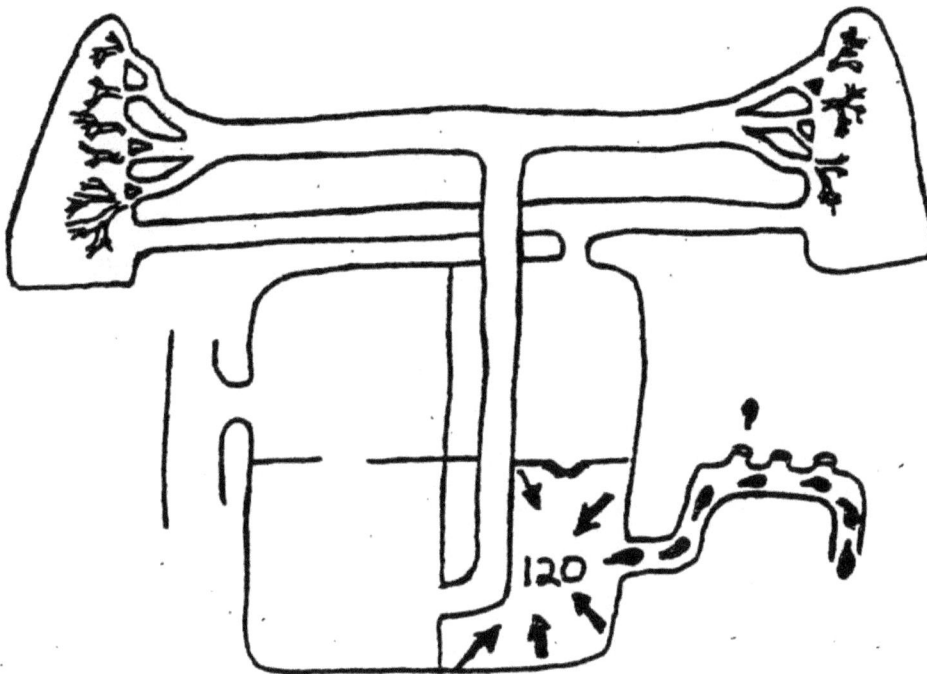

Aortic Insufficiency

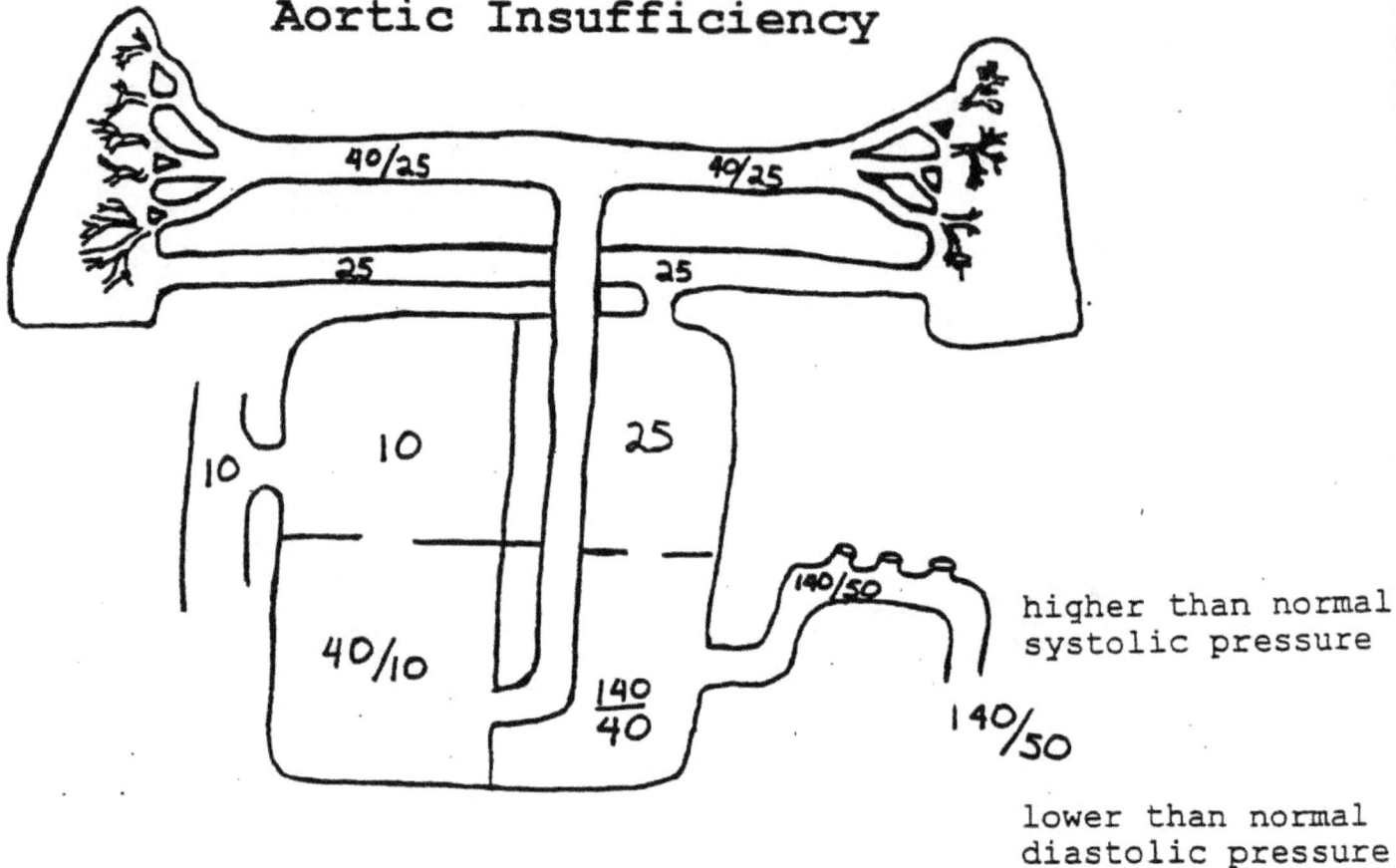

40/25   40/25

25   25

10   10   25

40/10   140/40

140/50

higher than normal systolic pressure

140/50

lower than normal diastolic pressure

Aortic insufficiency is a **leaky** aortic valve. Instead of blood in the aorta flowing into the vasculature, some of it leaks back into the left ventricle during ventricular diastole.

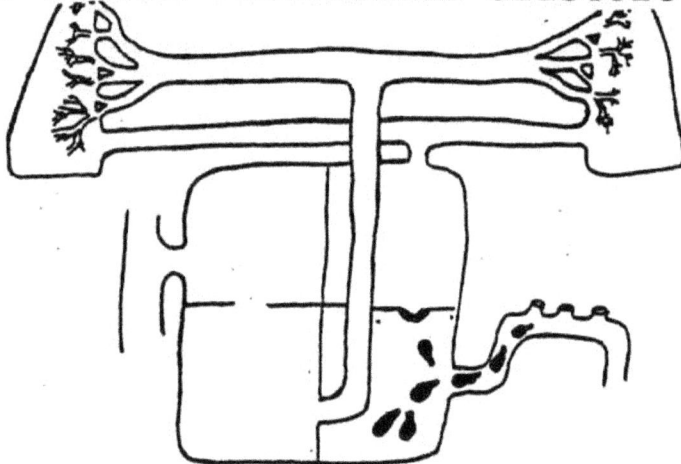

During diastole, when pressure is low in the left ventricle and the valve is closed, blood from the high-pressure aorta is leaking back into the left ventricle. This results in higher left ventricle diastolic pressure and lower aortic diastolic pressure.

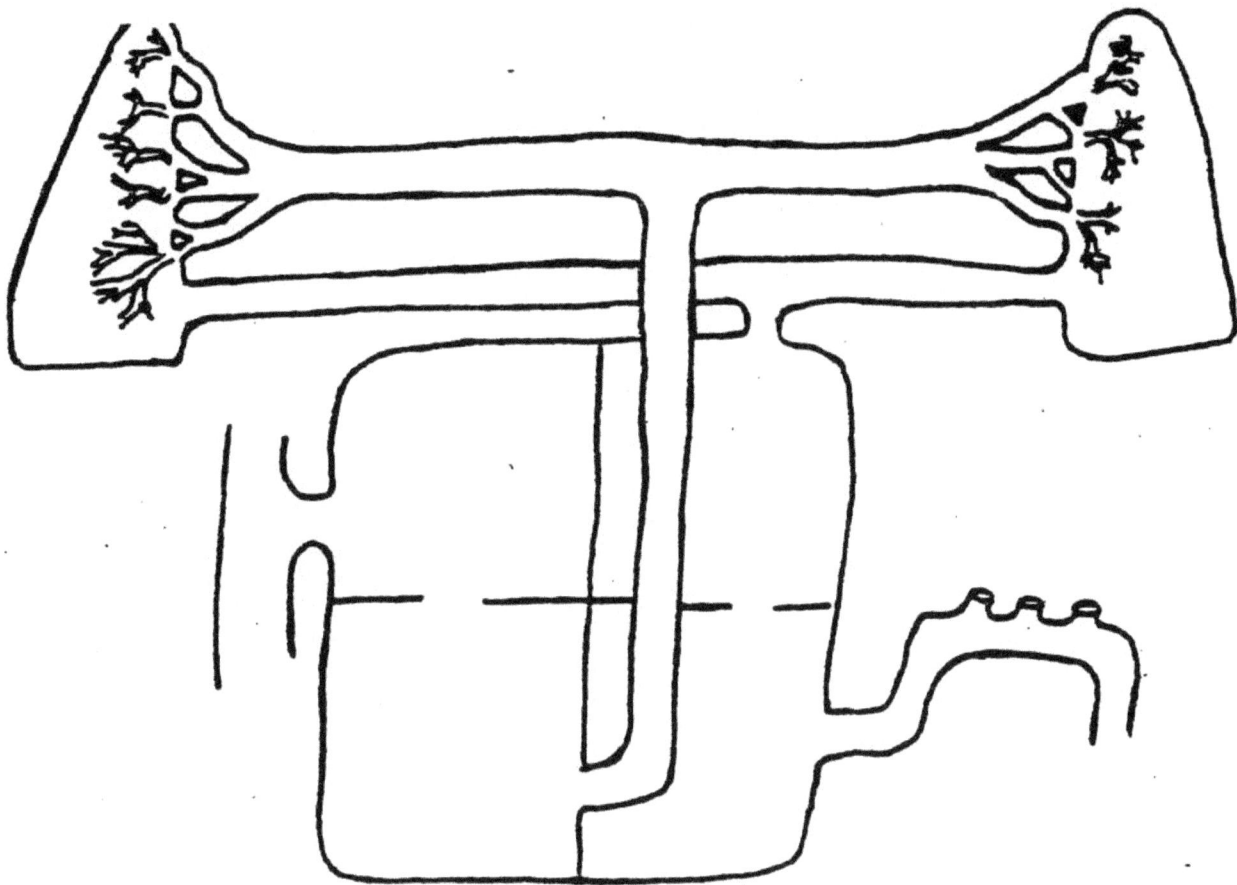

The left ventricle will become over distended from
high diastolic pressure.

In wide open aortic insufficiency, aortic diastolic
will be the same as left ventricular end diastolic
pressure because so much blood will have leaked
back from the aorta into the left ventricle so that
their pressure will have equilibrated by the end of
the diastolic period.

This could result in pulmonary edema because the high LVEDP results in left atrial pressure greater than 25mm Hg and can back up into the pulmonary veins, causing flooding of the pulmonary airways.

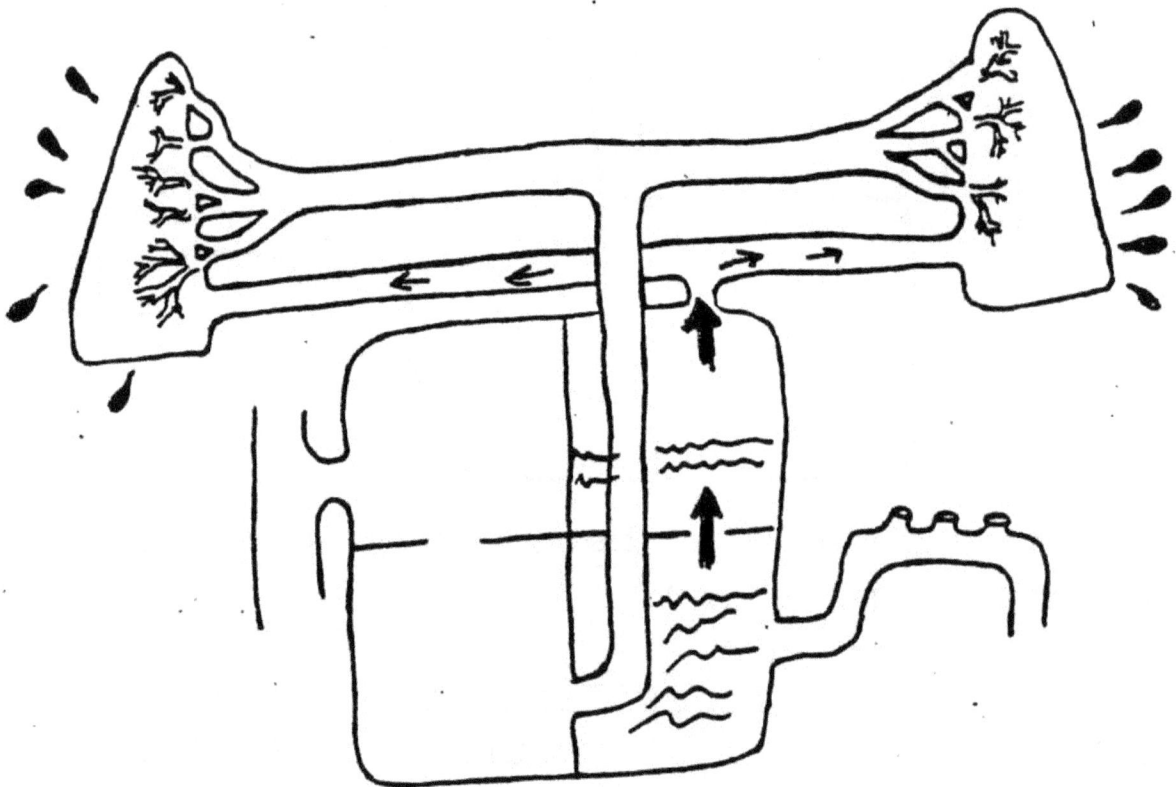

This back up will eventually result in right-sided failure when right atrial pressure exceeds 10mm Hg as a result of right ventricular strain and eventual failure.

MITRAL INSUFFICIENCY

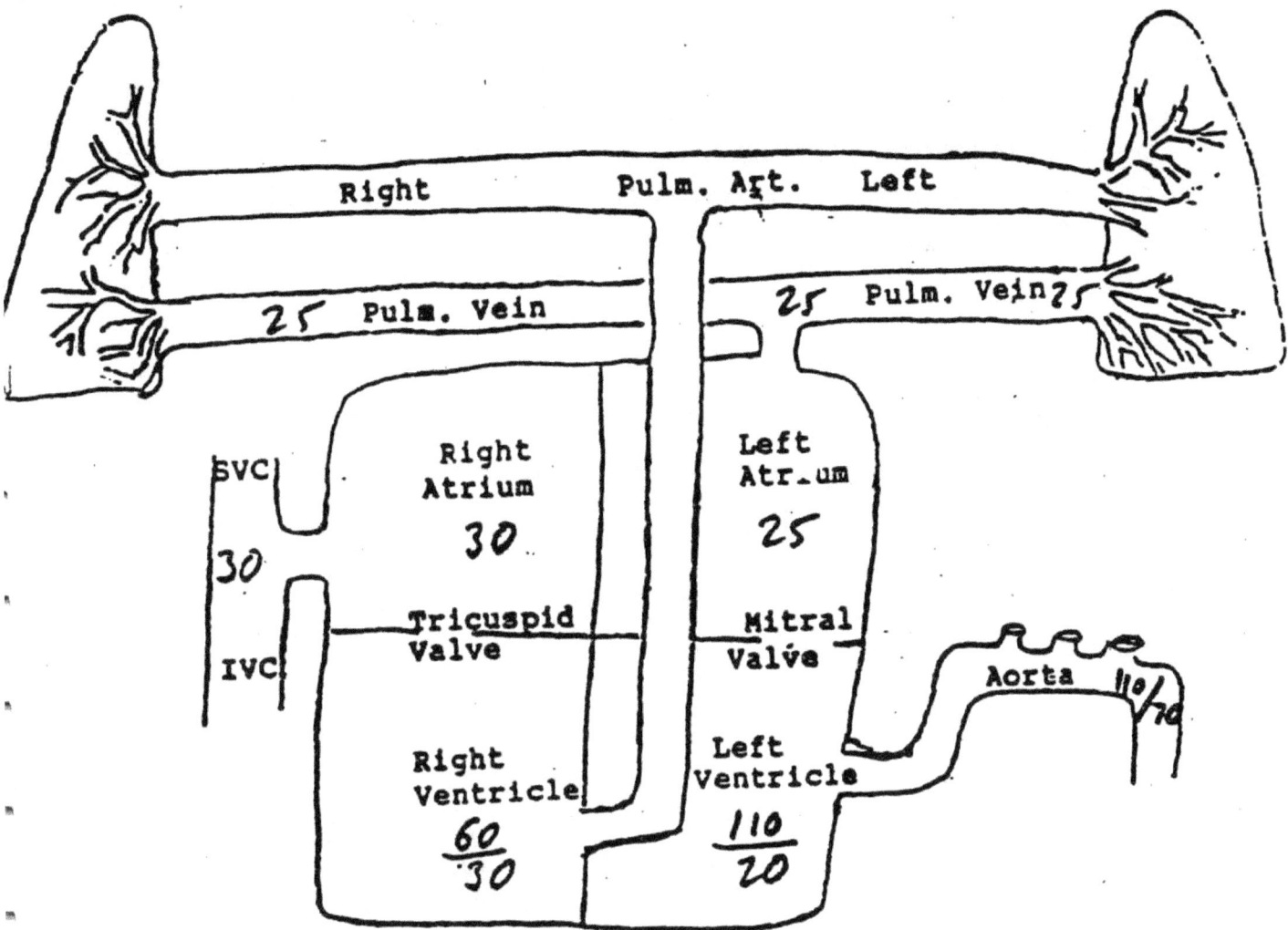

Like aortic insufficiency, in mitral valve
insufficiency, the mitral valve leaks. It is
usually caused by rheumatic fever. It is also
caused by mitral valve prolapse, where the valve
leaflets fall into the left atrium. Another cause
is coronary artery disease because ischemia of the
tissues of the left ventricle which surround the
mitral valve papillary muscles cause the mitral
leaflets not to contract properly during systole,
thus causing it to leak.

What happens is this: the left ventricle contracts.
Instead of all the blood going out of the aorta, some of it
leaks back to the left atrium. This can cause high left
atrial pressures, which can lead to pulmonary edema
(especially if the mitral regurgitation is sudden in
onset). In chronic mitral regurgitation, the left atrium
has time to stretch and can handle the regurgitant volume
without the left atrial pressure rising too much. This
protects the lungs from pulmonary edema.

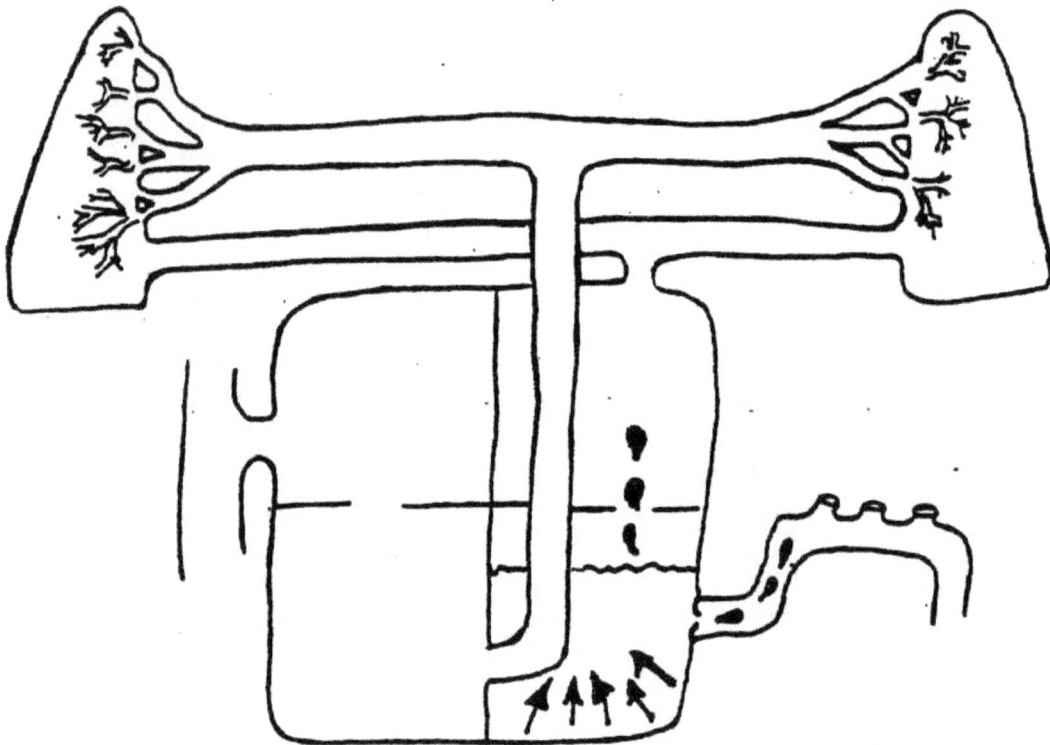

This causes an increase in left atrial pressure.
It also can lead to left ventricular failure since
it has to pump the regurgitated blood again on the
next beat, leading to high volume heart failure in
time.

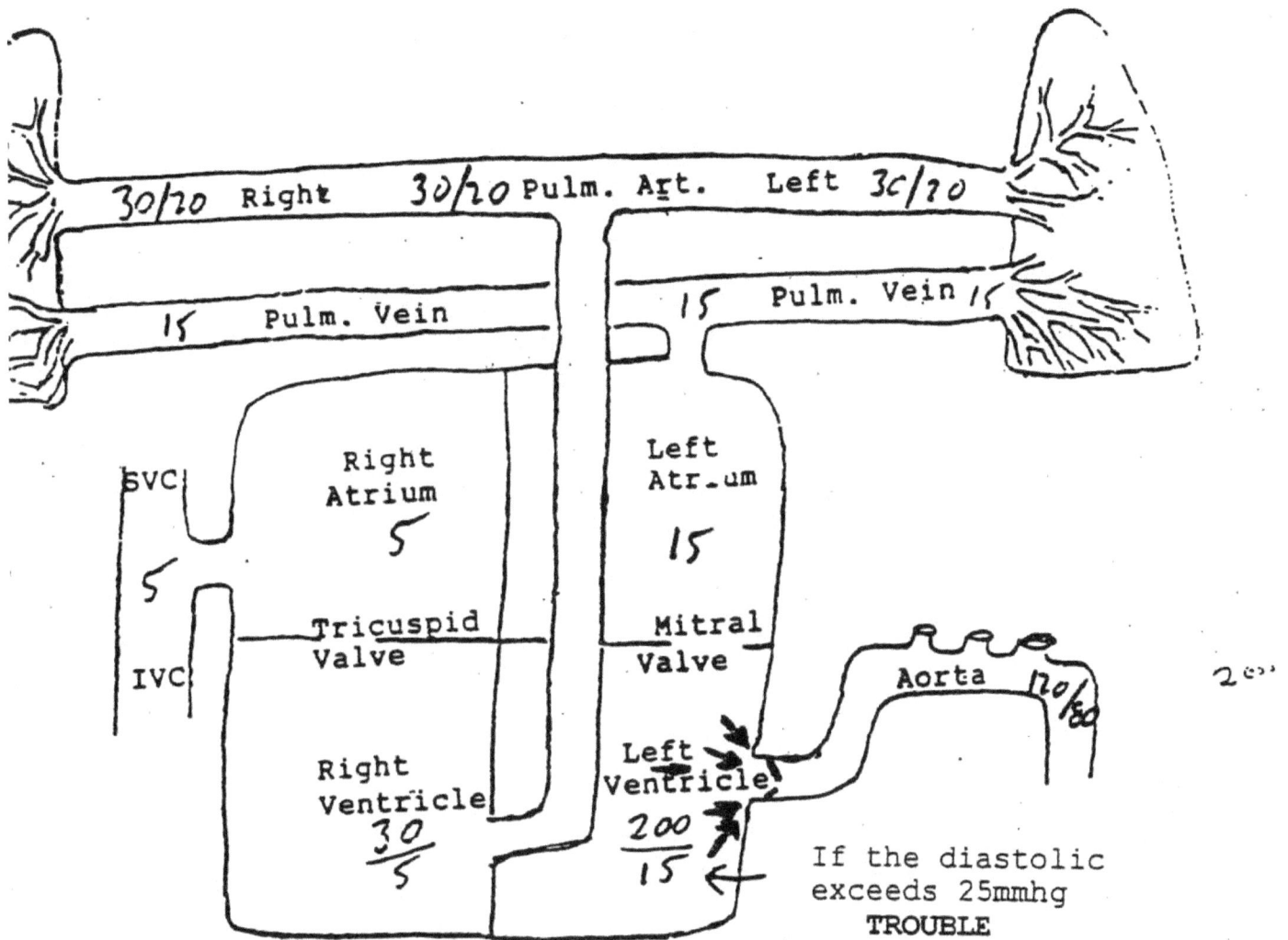

In aortic stenosis the aorta doesn't easily open. This is caused by calcification of the aortic valve and occasionally by rheumatic heart valve disease. The left heart has to contract more vigorously to generate enough pressure to overcome the resistance of the stenotic aortic valve.

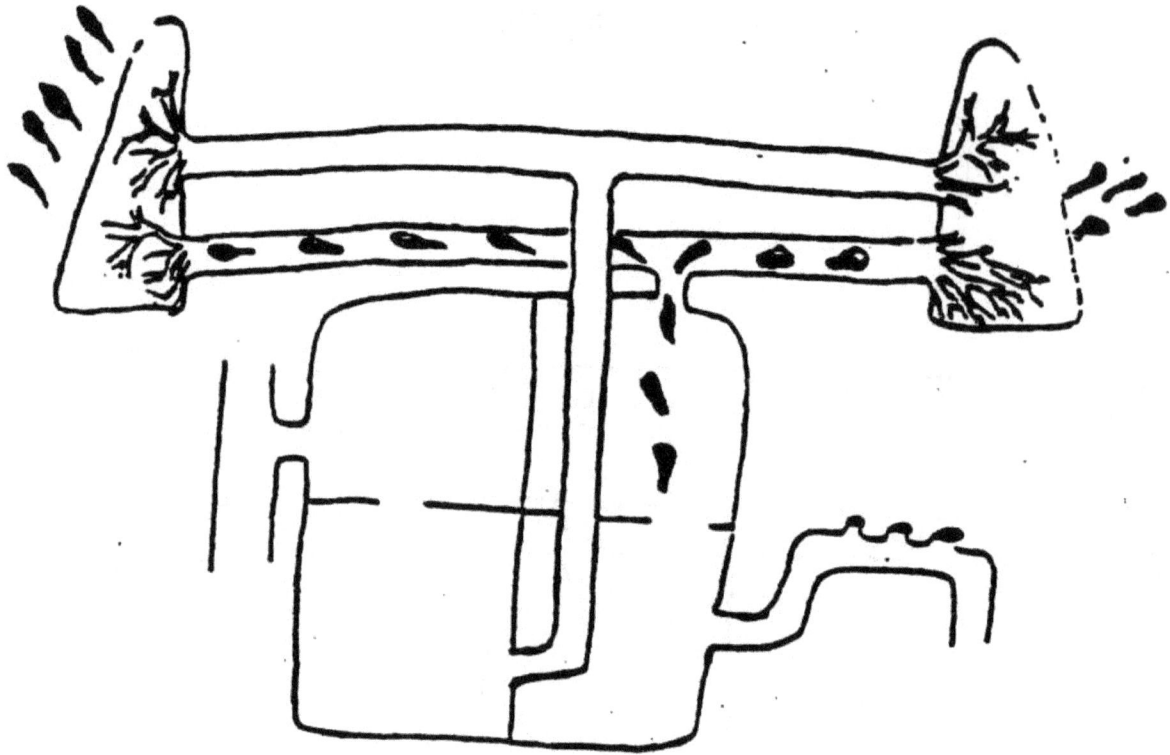

Working harder is good for your biceps. But when the heart works harder, the muscles not only enlarge (hypertrophy) but they stiffen as well. Since the walls don't stretch easily the diastolic pressure goes up rapidly and excessively as the left ventricle fills. You recall the sequence of events of the high pressure backing up through the lungs and further? That happens here, resulting in pulmonary edema.

Since the aortic valve is causing resistance, the left ventricular systolic is not the same as aortic systolic systolic pressure. A left hear catheterization or echocardiogram can measure aortic stenosis.

PULMONIC STENOSIS

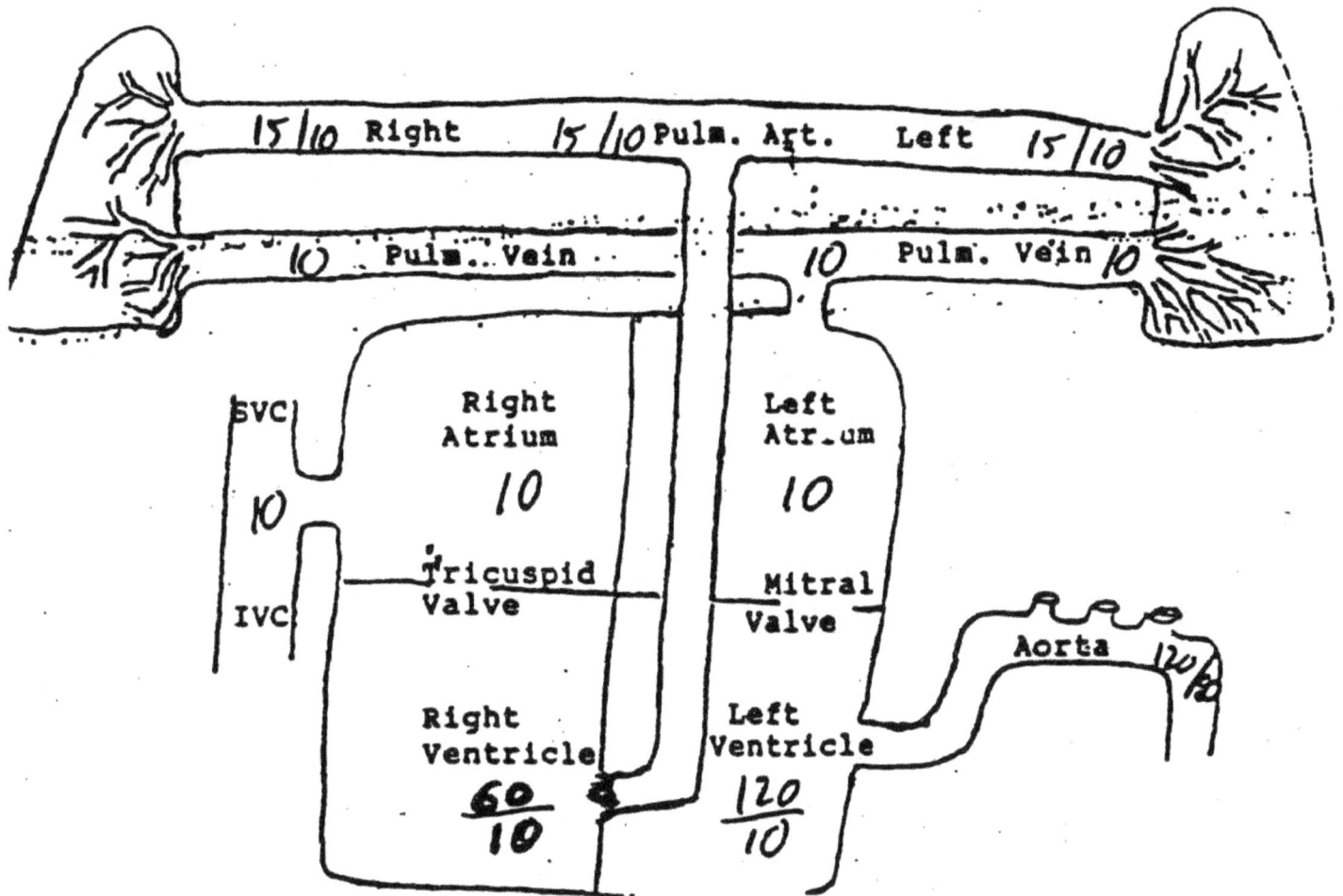

In pulmonary stenosis the pulmonary valve opens poorly or partially. You'll first notice normal pressures in the lungs and left side. The valve (stenotic valve) causes high pressures on the right side, which you see, are very elevated.

Having to work harder, the right ventricle becomes thicker (hypertrophy). After a long time, it dilates and balloons out which leads to right heart failure.

TRICUSPID STENOSIS

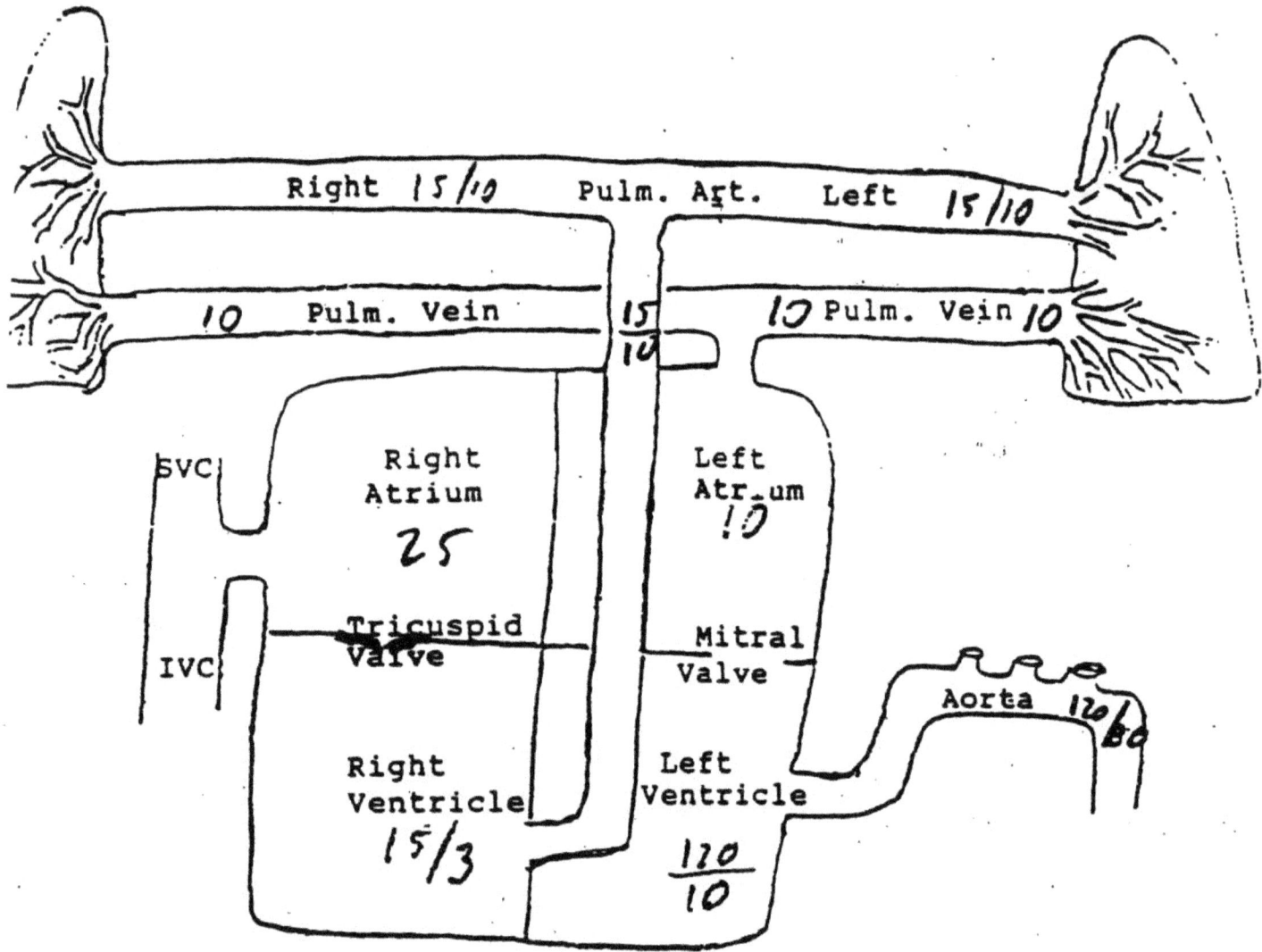

Right 15/10   Pulm. Art.   Left 15/10

10 Pulm. Vein   15/10   10 Pulm. Vein 10

SVC

Right Atrium
25

IVC

Tricuspid Valve

Right Ventricle
15/3

Left Atrium
10

Mitral Valve

Aorta 120/80

Left Ventricle
120/10

This shows up very clearly as elevated right atrial pressures.

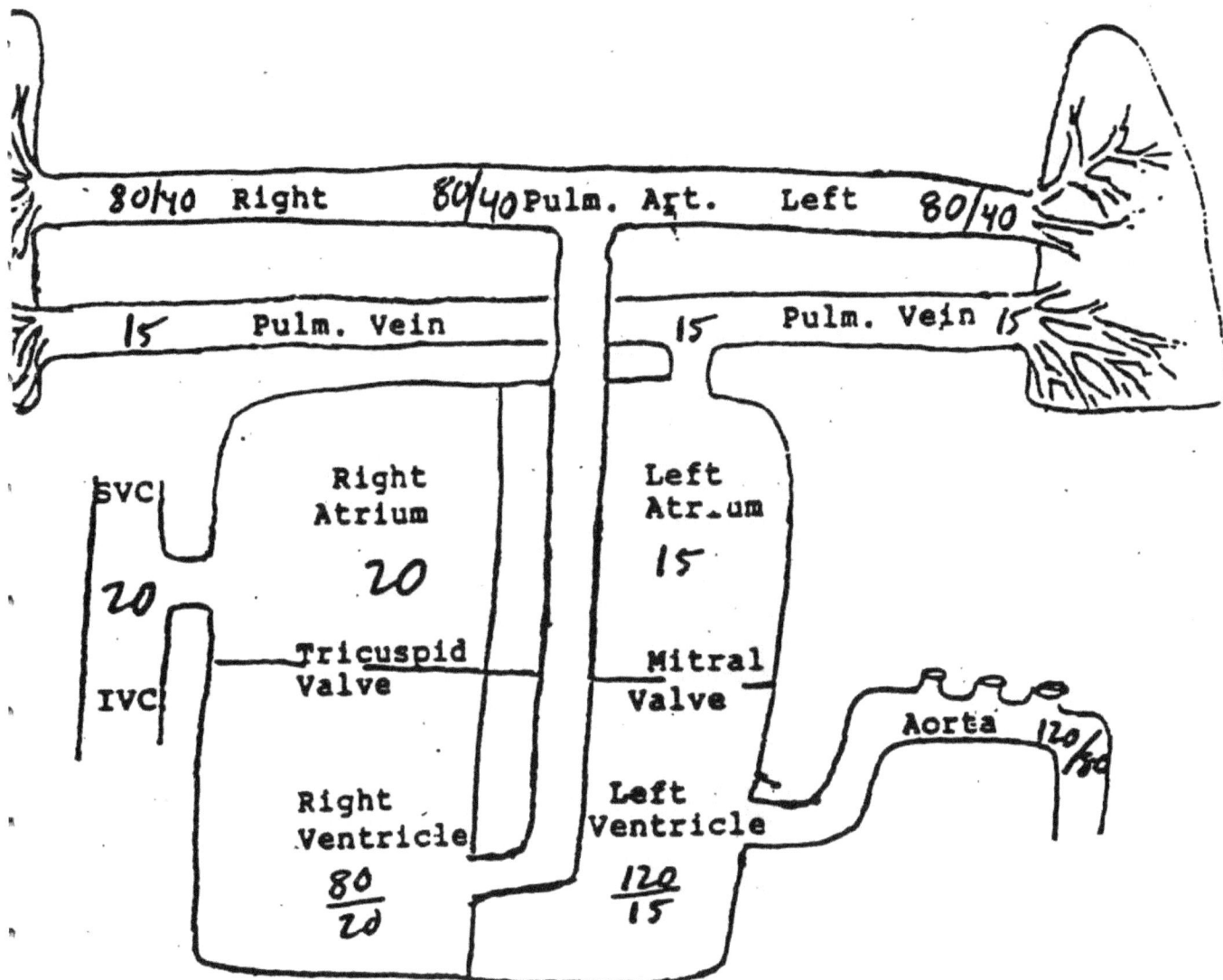

Diagram labels: 80/40 Right, 80/40 Pulm. Art., Left 80/40, 15 Pulm. Vein, 15, Pulm. Vein 15, SVC, 20, IVC, Right Atrium 20, Left Atrium 15, Tricuspid Valve, Mitral Valve, Aorta 120/80, Right Ventricle 80/20, Left Ventricle 120/15

This is right heart failure caused by lung disease like COPD or emphysema. In this situation, destruction of pulmonary capillaries causes increased congestion in the remaining capillaries. This is like way too many cars at rush hour on the interstate. It just slows down traffic. And the traffic congestion backs up for miles. You'll notice increases in pressure on the right side and normal pressures on the left side.

You can see high pressures in the pulmonary artery.

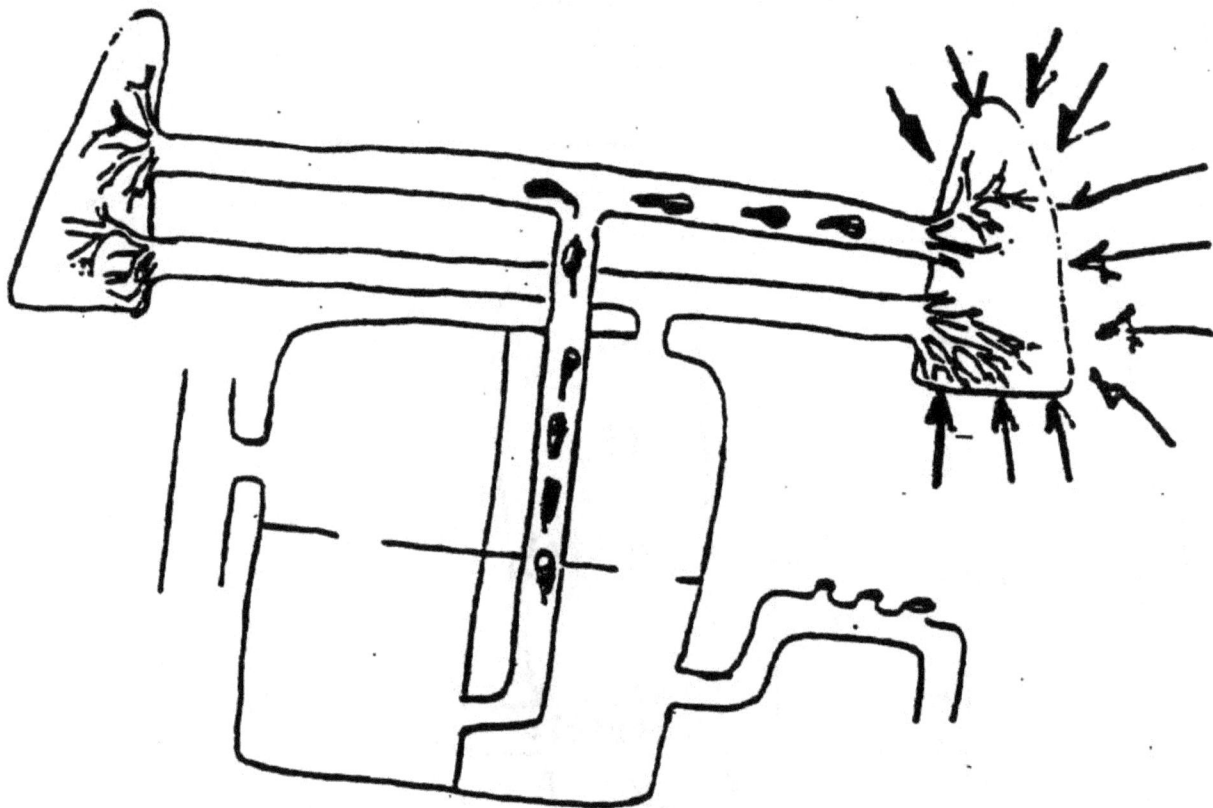

If high pulmonary artery pressure continues, it will lead to right ventricular failure. You know what that looks like - systemic venous hypertension pedal edema, distended jugular veins, ascites.

CONGESTIVE HEART FAILURE

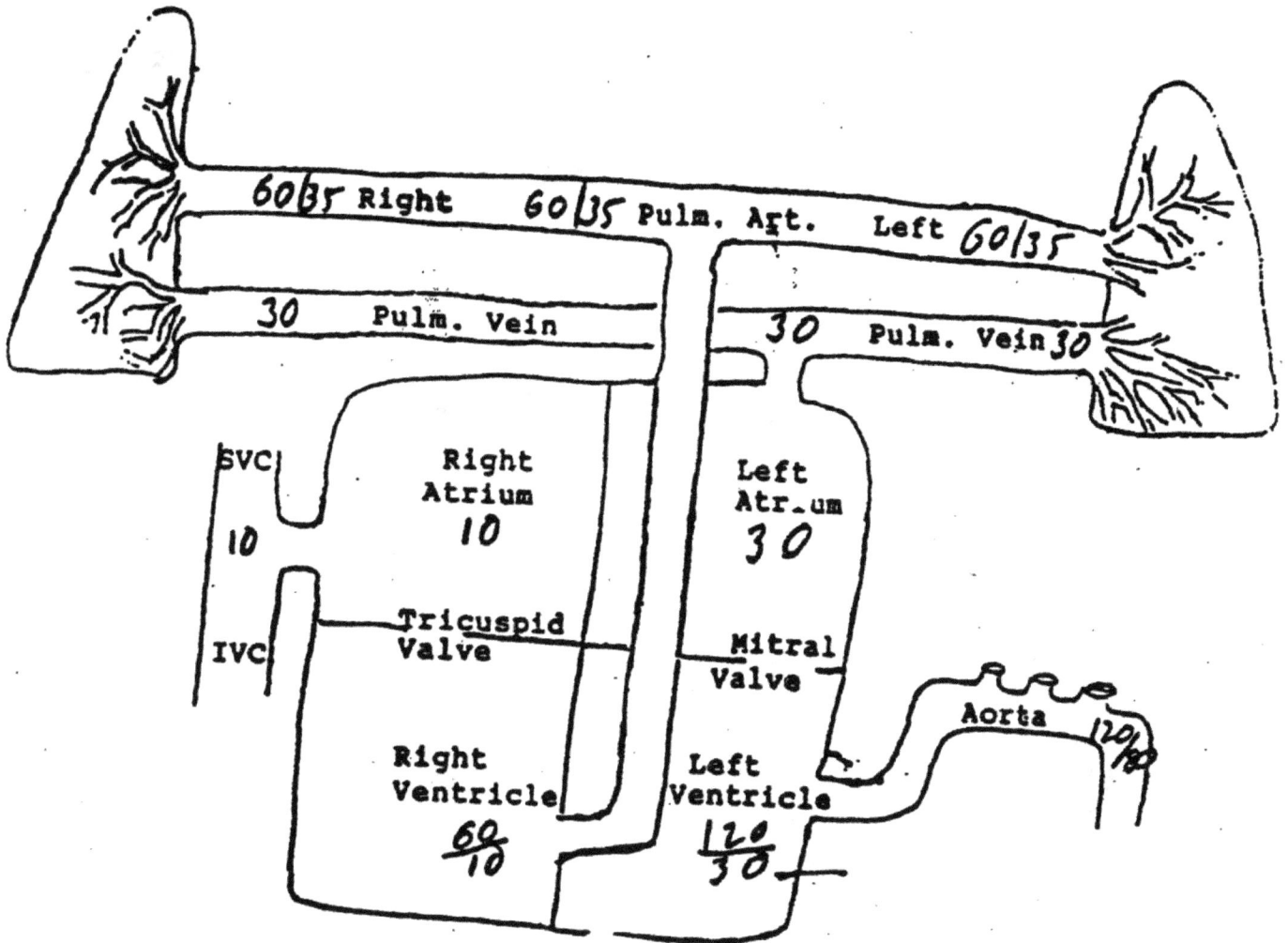

Congestive heart failure (CHF) is a weak heart -
usually from a previous heart attack. The heart
cannot pump blood as quickly and forcefully as it
should.

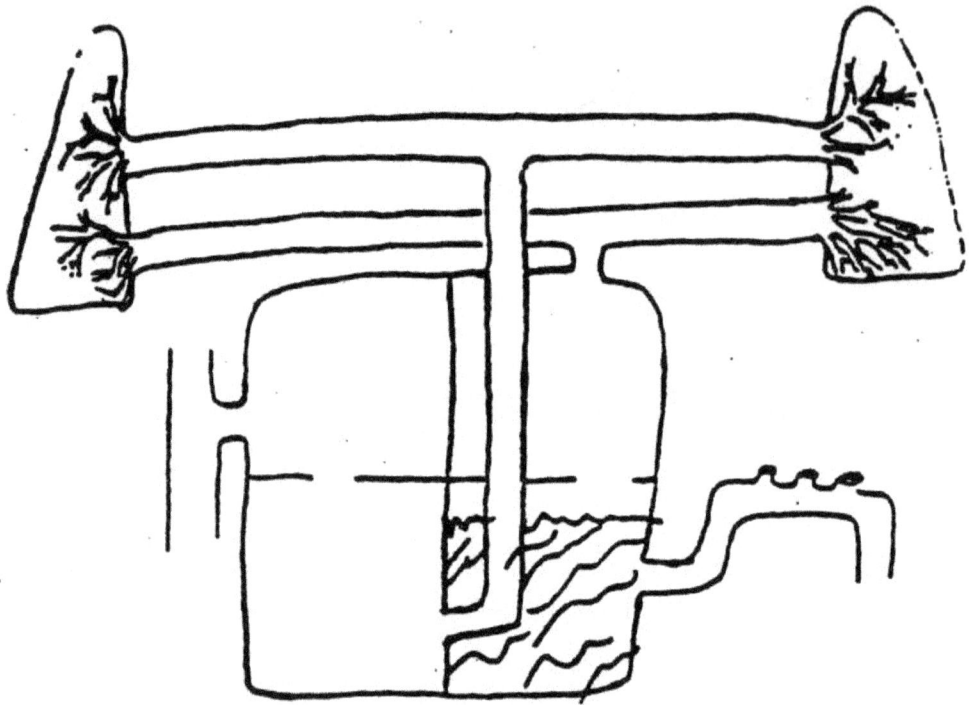

It compensates by filling more volume on each stroke (higher pre-load) and higher diastolic pressure. You see elevated left ventricular diastolic. The heart actually grows. It doesn't get larger muscles, it stretches. A dilated heart with a 30% ejection fraction will pump more volume of blood with each stroke. If it can only pump 30% of each stroke volume, then the left ventricle must contract many more times to pump enough blood.

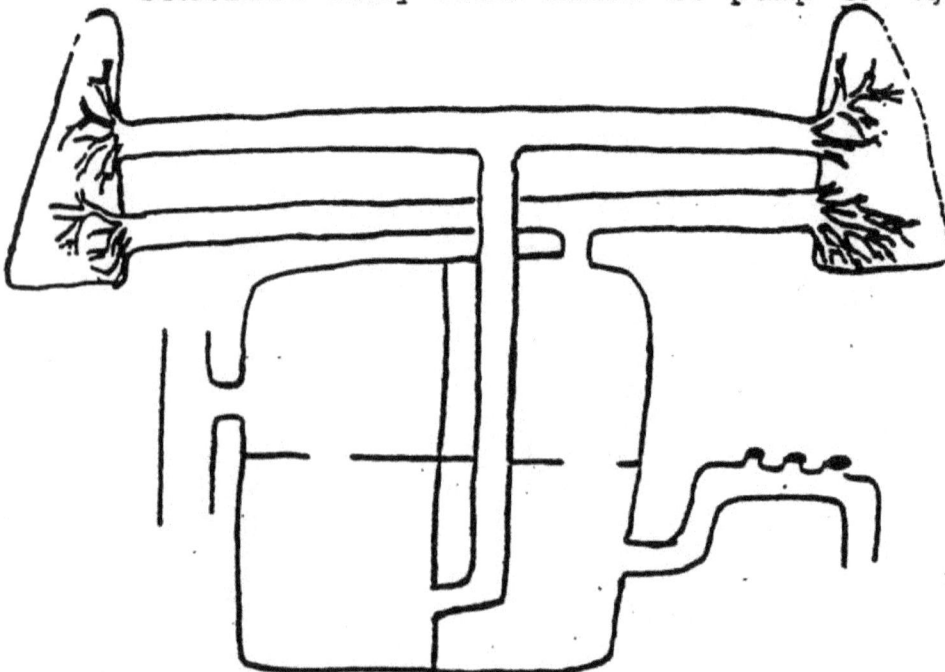

When left ventricular end diastolic reaches 25mm Hg, left
arterial pressure will also be 25. If left arterial
pressure is 25, the pressure will back up into the
pulmonary veins **and capillaries**

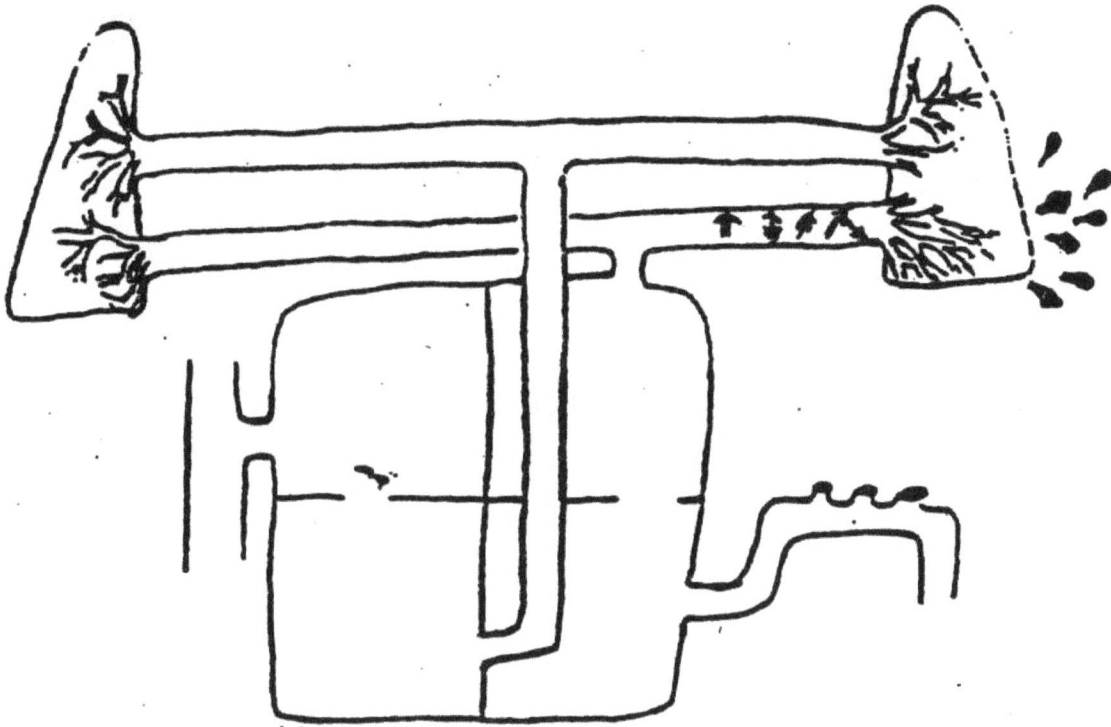

High pressure (more than 25mm Hg) in the pulmonary
capillaries will leak into the airways - flooding them with
fluid. This is called pulmonary edema. You recall that is
characterized by pink frothy sputum.

Another compensating mechanism is high systemic vascular
resistance. High resistance in the skeletal muscles, GI
tract, and renal vessels allows more blood to flow to the
brain when there isn't enough flow to go around. This
mechanism tends to work against the efficient functioning
of the heart due to the increase in systemic vascular
resistance (after load).

SHOCK

In shock the system blood pressure is low or the cardiac output is low. This causes insufficient blood supply to body tissues. There are three main causes: low blood volume, cardiogenic shock and septic shock.

SEPTIC SHOCK

In septic shock, there is a profound dilation of the arterioles and venules. This results from the gram negative germs in the blood stream. Don't ask why. Since all the blood is in the vasculatue, it doesn't make it back to the heart. The main difference between cardiogenic shock and volume loss is that the cardiac output is high in cardiogenic shock

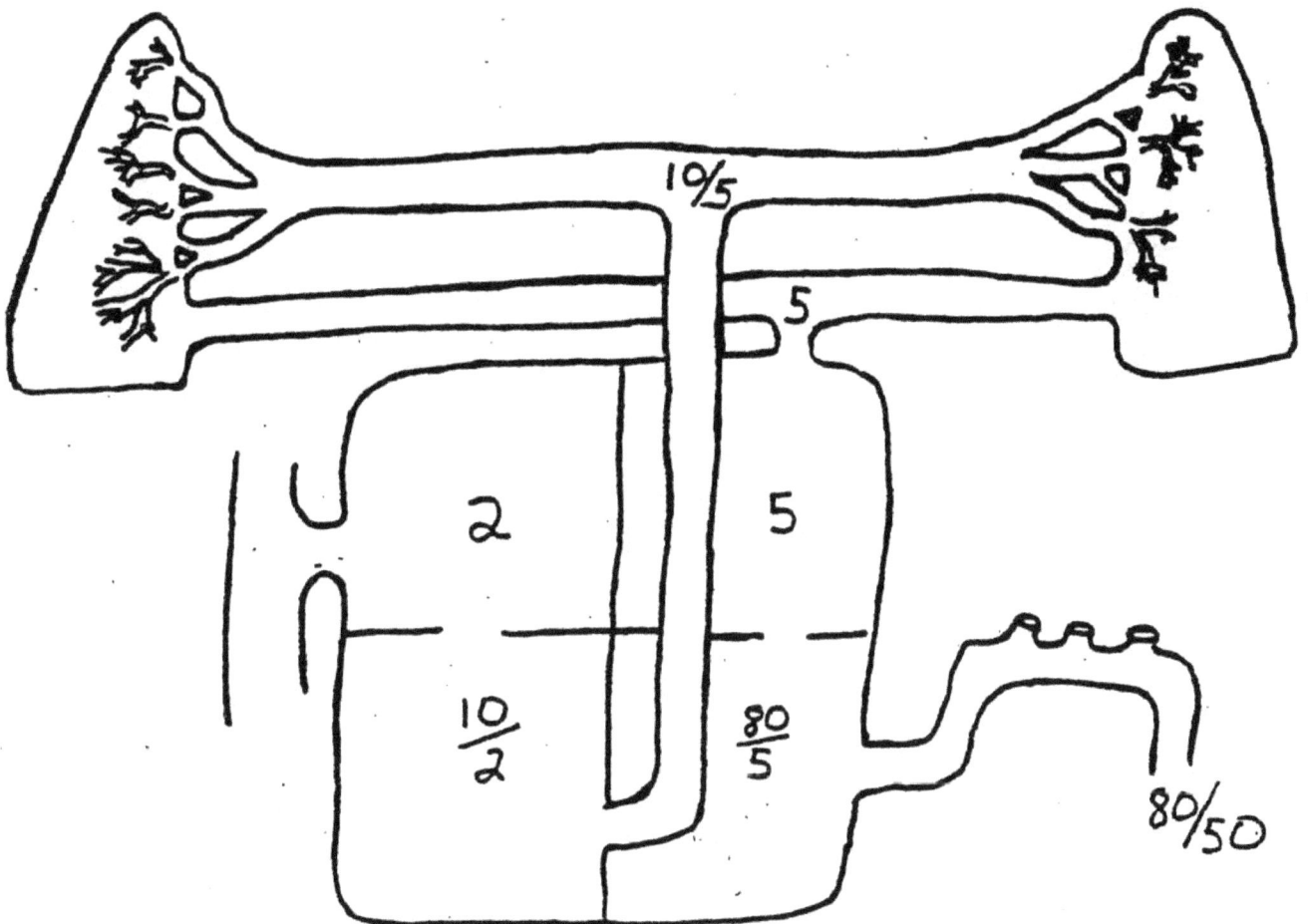

CARDIOGENIC SHOCK

Cardiogenic shock is the result of a weak heart. It is usually caused by myocardial infarction, cardiomyopathy or severe valvular disease. You'll notice a low left ventricular systolic. That's the best the weak heart can do.
You'll also notice a low systemic blood pressure.
The body reacts similarlyto volume loss here. It detects low cardiac output and vasoconstricts tomaintain circulation to the brain and heart. However the filling pressures
(left and right diastolic) are normal because the ventricles get enough blood they just can't eject it.

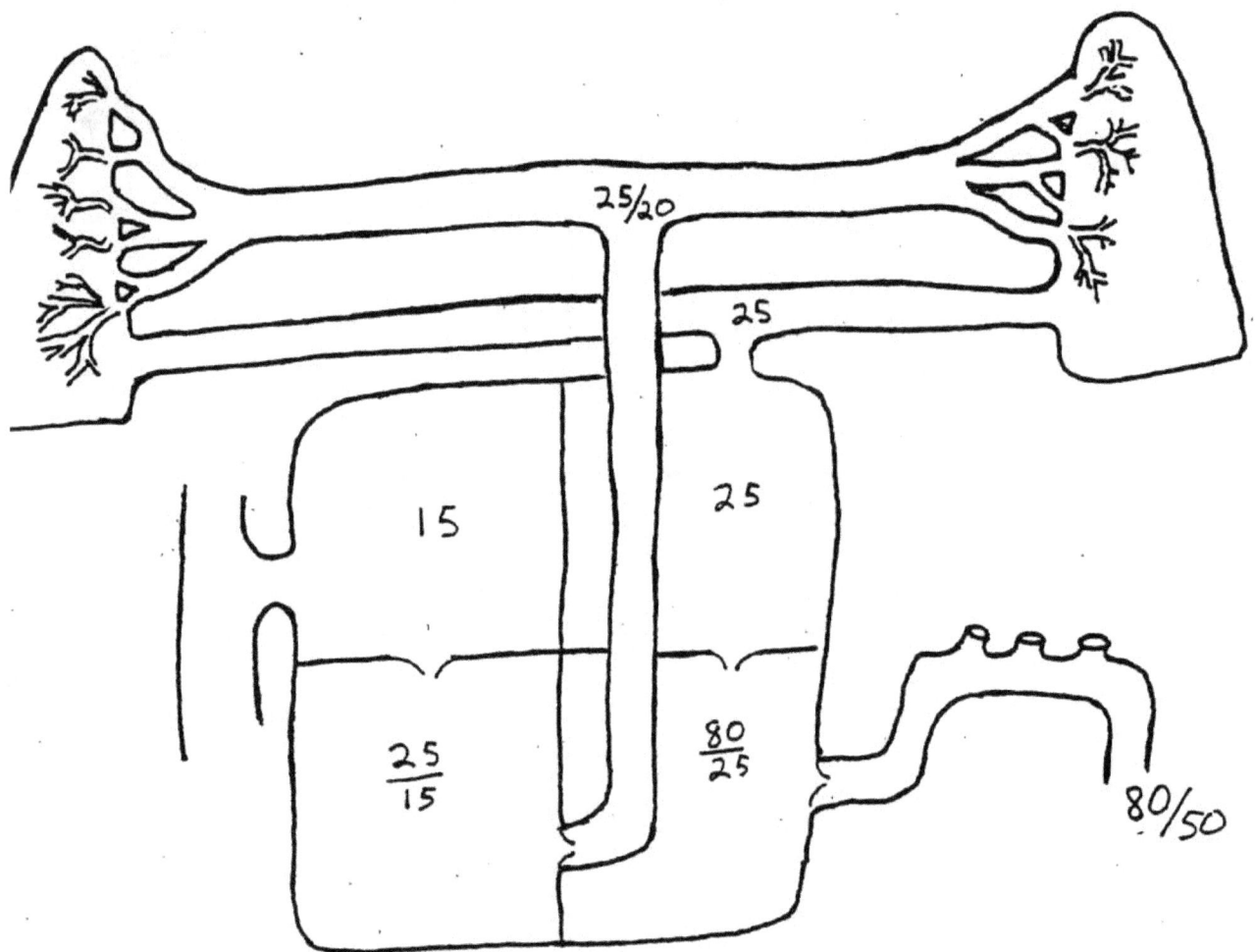

FLUID OVERLOAD

In the hospital setting, there are times when patients get too much fluid. Examples are blood trans fusion or excessive I.V. crystaloid infusion. This will lead to elevations in all the pressures on both sides of the heart, causing manefestations of both left and right heart failure - leg edema, distended jugular veins, pulmonary edema.

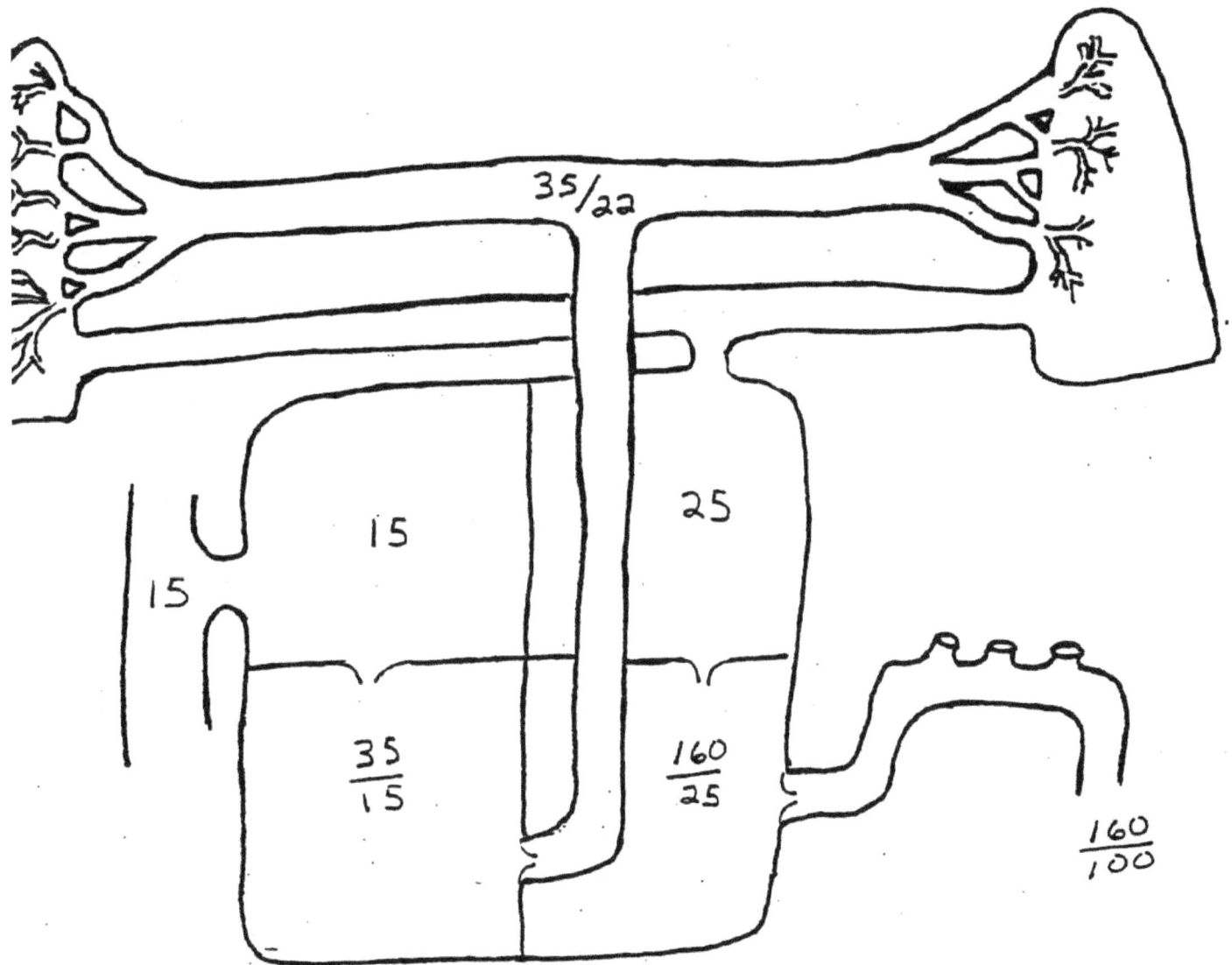

VOLUME LOSS

Fluid volume loss is caused by bleeding, dehydration, diarrhea, vomiting, insufficient fluid intake or excessive sweating. In volume loss, the body tries to maintain blood to the brain by clamping down on the blood flow to muscles, kidneys, G.I. tract and skin. This causes the classic signs of low urine output and cold clammy skin. On the diagram you'll notice low filling pressures (left and right ventricular diastolic) because there is just no blood. The left ventricle is pumping what little blood is there. So the left ventricular systolic is lower. Even though the systemic blood pressure looks low, its actually higher than it would have been with out the systemic vascular contraction.

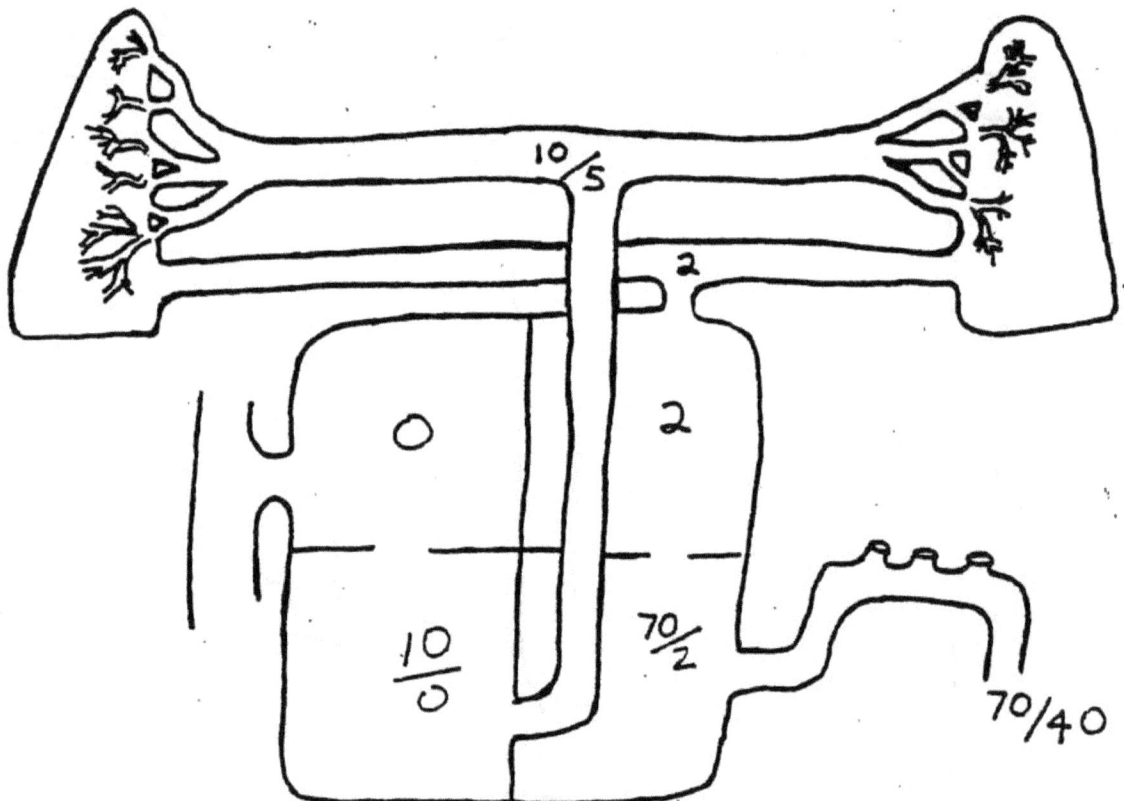

MEDICAL JOKES

Cardiac Joke: What do you get when you spill a urinal?
Answer: see bottom of page

Immunology Joke: "I'm allergic to lasix. It makes me pee."

Hematology Joke: A vampire goes into a blood bank and asks for one unit of packed red cells and one unit of fresh frozen plasma. The phlebotomist yells back to the tech, "Gimme a Blud and a Blud Lite."

Otolaryngology Joke. For otitis media the doctor ordered "corticosporin drops in the R ear QID" The pharmacist called back to say corticosporin doesn't come in suppository form.

Orthopedic Joke (told by an infectious disease doctor): What do you need to do to pass the orthopedic boards? Be able to bench 200 pounds and spell Ancef.

Urology Joke: The doctor is doing a prostate exam. The guy yells, "That hurts!"
The doctor says," I'm using two fingers."
"Why?"
"I want a second opinion."

Infectious Disease Joke: How do you get a Kleenex to dance? Put a little boogie in it.

C.V. Joke: Did you hear about the two red blood cells who loved in vein?

To impress someone try saying, a gram of acetaminocin instead of two extra strength Tylenols.

G.I. Cartoon: There is a doctor, a nurse and a patient. The patient is draped and in the jack knife position presumabley for a sigmoidoscopy.. The nurse is holding a tray with a bottle of beer. The doctor with an angry look says, "No, I said I wanted a butt light."

I.C.U. Cartoon: There is a patient in an I.C.U. bed with monitors, dynamaps, oxygen, and all the familiar paraphanalia. He is talking on the phone saying, "Bells are ringing and the T.V.has a straight line."

A guy goes in to see a doctor. He touches his head and says, every time I touch it here it hurts." He touches his stomach and says the same thing. He touches his knee and repeats it again. The doctor examines him and says, "Your finger is broken."

Answer to cardiology joke: You get a Pee Wave

A very attractive young man and a vivacious young lady meet in a fashionable night club and they hit it off immediately. Later in the evening they discuss spending the night together and leave immediately for the woman's apartment. As they are getting ready for bed the woman goes into the bathroom and starts to compulsively wash her hands for an excessive length of time. The man asks, "Are you a doctor?"

"Yes."

"Don't tell me! A surgeon! Right?"

"Yes. How did you know?"

"It was obvious. I could see your concern for transmitting germs and preventing infection."

They go have sex and afterward, the woman asks the man, "Are you a doctor?"

"Yes."

"Don't tell me! An anesthesiologist! Right?"

"Yes. How did you know?"

"I didn't feel a thing."

Ophthalmology Joke: This takes place in a very exclusive private girls' school. The eighth grade science teacher, Mr. Johnson, asks, " What organ of the body, when stimulated, expands to six times its normal size? Miss Smith?"

"Mr. Johnson, I don't think that is a proper question to ask a girl of my age and social standing."

He calls on another student, "Miss Jones?"

"The pupil of the eye"

"That is correct. Miss Smith I have three things to say to you. One: you didn't do your homework. Two: you have a dirty mind. Three: someday you are going to be very disappointed."

Orthopedic Joke. A guy sees a doctor. He says, "Everywhere I touch it hurts." He touches his forehead and says, "It hurts." He touches his stomach and says the same thing. He touches his knee. Again, same thing. The doctor says, "Let me examine you." After a few minutes of poking and prodding, "Your finger is broken."

Ask any surgeon to name the three best surgeons in the world. They'll have a hard time thinking of the other two.

"Do you know the definition of "innuendo"?

"Yeah sure. That's simple"

```
   explanatory of the text
²innuendo also inuendo \"\ n, pl innuendos or innuendoes
   1 : veiled, oblique, or covert allusion to something not directly
   named : HINT, INSINUATION (glossy fantasy, stylishness,
   naughty ~ —Time) (a talk punctuated with ~s on both
   sides —J.T.Farrell); esp : veiled or equivocal allusion re-
   flecting upon the character, ability, or other trait of the
   person referred to (try to undermine him by ~ —Kiplinger
   Washington Letter) (how difficult it is to set up a proper
   defense against ~ —M.S.Watson) (anonymous accusations,
   rumors, ~s —Nathan Schachner)  2 : a parenthetical ex-
   planation of the text of a legal document; esp : an interpreta-
   tion in a pleading of expressions alleged to be injurious or
   libelous
³innuendo also inuendo \"\ vb -ED/-ING/-S [²innuendo] vi
```

"No. It's an Italian enema."

Plastic Surgery: During routine surgery a woman goes into cardiac arrest. After superhuman efforts and being apparently dead she miraculously recovers. During this ordeal she has an out-of-body experience in which she talks to God. God tells her she has forty more years to live and she should make the most of it be striving to be her best. From that she concludes she should improve her appearance and has liposuction, breast augmentation and a face lift. As she is leaving the hospital a bus hits her and instantly kills her. When she gets to heaven she asks God," What's this all about? You said..." God interrupts, "I didn't recognize you."

Surgery: How does a surgeon change a light bulb? They Just hold it in the socket and stand still. The earth revolves around them.

Psychiatry: How many psychiatrists does it take to change a light bulb? Only one. But first, the light bulb has to want to change.

A man on a crowded bus a man sees a woman with grocery bags and two small children. He gets up to give her his seat and helps her with the bags.
"Thank you. You're sweet" she says.
"I know. I'm diabetic."
Thanks to Dr. Murray Miller, an endocrinologist, for that one.

How do you tell the difference between an oral thermometer and a rectal thermometer? The taste.

Why did the cookie go to the doctor? It was feeling crummy.

An internist, a psychiatrist, a surgeon and a pathologist are duck hunting. The internist sees something moving in the trees. He says to the psychiatrist, "Is that a duck?" The psychiatrist says, "It's a duck if it thinks it's a duck." The surgeon grabs his shot gun, BAM BAM BAM and says to the pathologist, "Tell me if that is a duck."

Do you have any good, clean medical jokes? If you do, please send it to me. If I include it on this list, I will give you a copy of any one of my books. Also please specify whether you want your name included as the contributor – or would like to remain anonymous. Please send jokes to Malcolm Rosenberg, P.O. Box 770793, Coral Springs FL 33077 and tell me which book you want. Simplified Arterial Blood Gases, Simplified Ventilators, Simplified Hemodynamics, Drug Calculations for Nurses Who Hate Numbers, or Making the Patients Laugh.

Q: Why are barracuda and sharks so healthy?
A: They eat fish.

Q: What is the cause of inverted P-waves?
A: Hypospadia

Q: What is the therapeutic effect of mixing Rogaine and Viagra?
A: Don King

A busy urologist's office answers the phone, "Urology Associates. Can you hold?"

Q: What did the epididymis say to the seminal vesicle?
A: "There is a vas deferens between us"

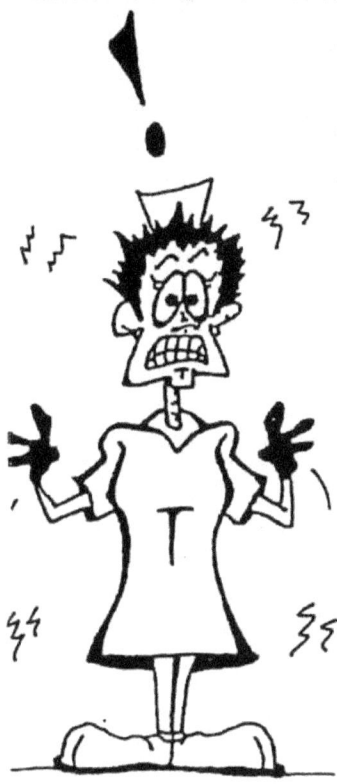
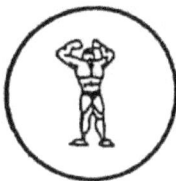 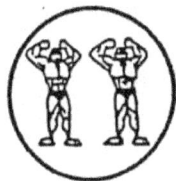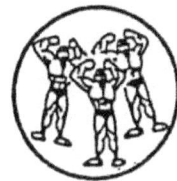
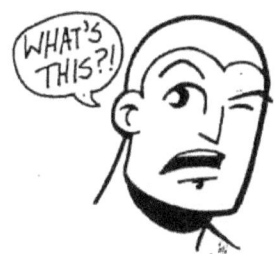

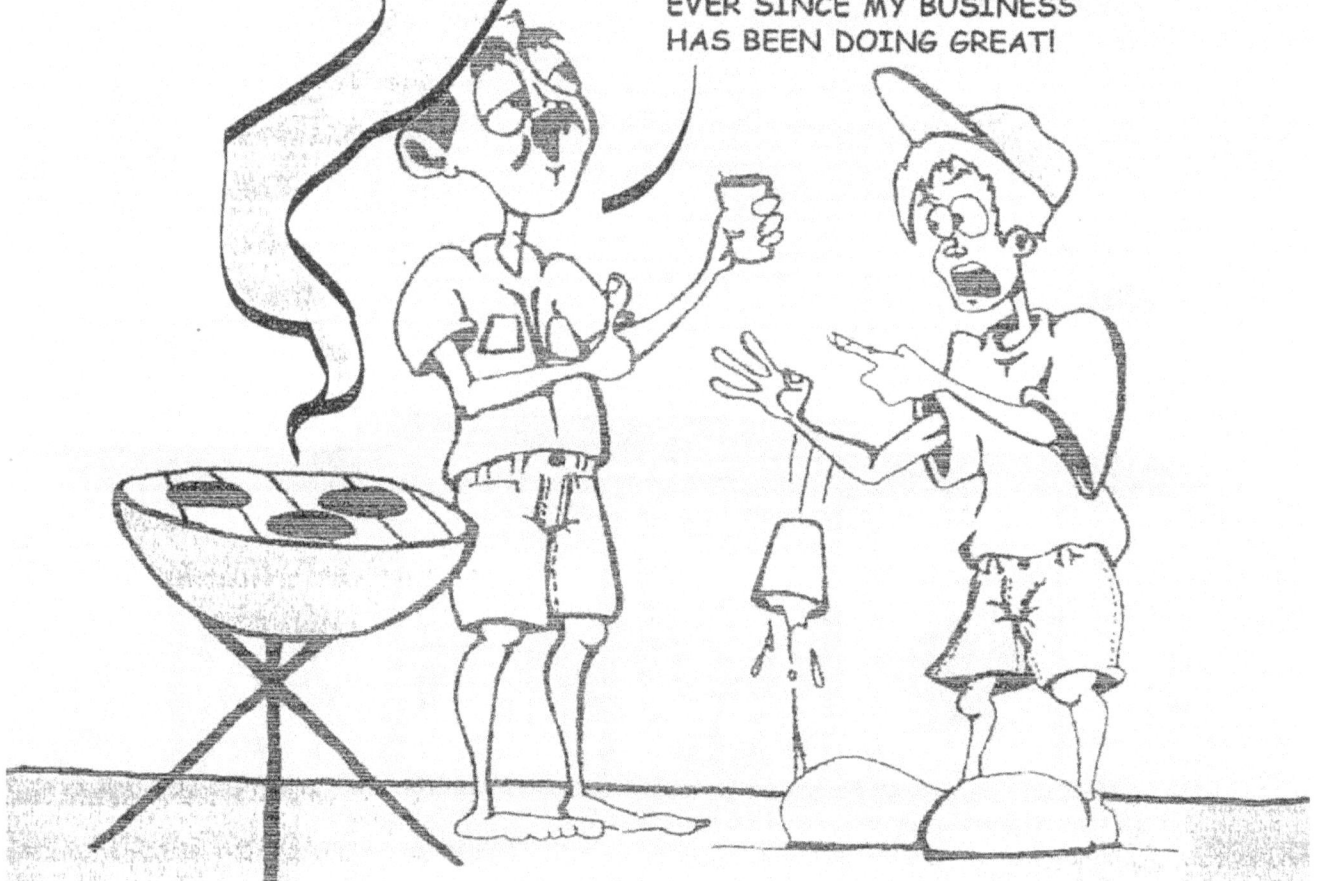

Simplified Hemodynamics ©1999

Retail: $11.95

ISBN 0-9725483-3-5

9780972548335

0 700814 498016

7 00814 49801 6